Age and Vulnerability

A guide to better care

Professor Olive Stevenson, MA (Oxon)

Head of School of Social Studies and
Department of Social Work,
University of Nottingham

With a chapter by
Michael Key, BA, MA

Edward Arnold
A division of Hodder & Stoughton
LONDON   MELBOURNE   AUCKLAND

Age Concern handbooks

Also published in this Series:

Counselling Older People: A creative response to ageing
Steve Scrutton

© 1989 Olive Stevenson

First published in Great Britain 1989
Reprinted 1990

British Cataloguing in Publication Data

Stevenson, Olive
    Age and vulnerability: a guide to better care.—
    (Age Concern handbooks).
    1. Old persons. Care
    1. Title   II. Key, Michael   III. Series
    362.6

    ISBN 0-340-48670-8

Whilst the advice and information in this book is believed to be true
and accurate at the date of going to press, neither the author nor the
publisher can accept any legal responsibility or liability for any errors or
omissions that may be made.

Typeset in 10/11 pt Cheltenham Light by Colset Pte Ltd, Singapore
Printed and bound in Great Britain for Edward Arnold,
a division of Hodder & Stoughton Limited, Mill Road, Dunton Green,
Sevenoaks, Kent TN13 2YA by Biddles Ltd, Guildford and King's Lynn

Contents

Foreword

David Hobman

Two years before becoming Chairman of Age Concern England in 1980, Olive Stevenson addressed a conference of the movement in Harrogate. The title of her paper was 'Ageing – a Professional Perspective'.

In her conclusions to a presentation which both moved and excited her audience, Olive Stevenson described the values which she suggested should be the basis of our work with and for older people.

These included the need to search for ways which would enable old people to give as well as to receive; to maintain family ties through the establishment of a partnership between carers and the wider community; and to develop an understanding of the variable nature of dependence in old age, as a prerequisite for the provision of appropriate help. In the application of our special skills and knowledge, if we are involved in the caring process, we must recognise that we may each be called upon to *do*, but also in a psychological sense to stay with a person who is troubled, restless or fearful because this is how we affirm the value of the relationship.

This emphasis on the need to apply the skills and values of social work to older people, coupled with the imperative to raise the level of interest and enthusiasm of working with them, by recognising that there are genuine professional satisfactions to be derived from the task, gave a new impetus to Olive Stevenson's audience at a time when the Age Concern movement was itself evolving its own strategies for care.

These have now been codified and enshrined in a regular publication of a handbook which is produced every three years.

Olive Stevenson's address in Harrogate, and her subsequent leadership in the Chair between 1980 and 1983, came at a critical period for Age Concern when we were in the process of working out how to apply the principles we had established some years earlier in the publication of the manifesto on the place of older people in our society.

The manifesto had stressed the importance of personal autonomy and choice from a range of genuine options as the basis of a full life in a democratic society.

The manifesto also suggested that enlightened self-interest is the most powerful motivating force for social change. Historically this has always been the case. It could clearly be seen in the development of the infant welfare clinics half a century ago as well as in the broader educational context itself.

What we needed then was help in applying the principles enshrined in a global statement about desirable objectives which we could share in the abstract, but which needed practical application.

At the same time, we were beginning to campaign actively, in association with others, to persuade more people involved in the health and social services to consider the reasonable claims of older people to enjoy the best skills they had to offer, and to understand the intellectual challenge involved in seeking solutions to their difficulties. Whilst older people may have commanded a larger portion of the budget of the social service departments, very little professional time was applied to their care.

Olive Stevenson's involvement with Age Concern was important at that time for at least two reasons. Firstly, because she has the true gifts of a communicator, able to share her understanding of what are often complex human needs and responses with lay audiences in terms they can interpret and work on, in the context of their daily lives. Secondly, as a distinguished teacher of social work and social policy, whose previous career had been more closely concerned with children, her identification with work with older people in general, and of Age Concern England in particular, provided a very significant symbolic message at a time when ageing was still fighting to find its way onto the agenda.

We still have a long way to go before Schools of Social Work or Medicine automatically have sufficient time in their curricula devoted to the subject, but there are other courses as well, where the challenge of later life should reflect a central theme. They range from nursing to architecture, or from transport management to theology, because, of course, they reflect universal issues of human life for all of us. But, if the teaching is to make a lasting impact, there is a continuing and growing need for literature designed to capture students' imagination when they are beginning to consider career options.

This is why I was so delighted when Olive Stevenson accepted an invitation, following her period of Chairmanship, and whilst I was still Director of Age Concern England, to write this book. It is also why I am grateful to my successor, Sally Greengross, for making it possible for me to write a brief foreword as a continuing expression of my belief that the social challenge of ageing is amongst the most important and interesting of our time, for both scholars and practitioners.

For some older people, and their families, later life has become a greater burden than it need be because of our failure to either understand the nature of the difficulties which older people have to overcome, or to provide for them properly. We also often fail to see that their problems can be as much a reflection of our own lack of concern, or readiness to respond with skill and imagination, as due to any inherent disabilities within the universal process of ageing itself.

Olive Stevenson shows us the way forward in recognition that our concern is with our own lives and our future, as much as it is with other people's.

Storrington, 1987   David Hobman

Acknowledgements

I am grateful to Professor Tom Arie for his helpful comments, to Sue Walton who generously shared her dissertation material on drug usage with me, and to Cherrylyn Senior who raised my awareness of the needs of black elderly people. Michael Key showed infinite patience in the drafting of his chapter and was generous in entrusting it to this book. My secretary, Ros Taylor, was unfailingly reliable in typing and retyping in a great hurry.

I owe a debt to David Hobman who made all this possible, and to Sally Greengross as well, from both of whom I have learnt much.

To them all, and Christine who has supported me behind the scenes in the endeavour – thank you.

This book is dedicated to my Aunt Hilda, who has taught me all through my life but especially in her old age. From her, I have learnt that it is possible to use the pain of loss constructively, to remain open to new relationships and to go on growing, intellectually and emotionally, throughout life.

About Age Concern

Age Concern England, the co-publishers of this book as well as a wide range of others, provides training, information and research for use by retired people and those who work with them. It is a registered charity dependent on public support for the continuation of its work.

The three other national Age Concern Organisations – Scotland, Wales and Northern Ireland together with Age Concern England – form a network of over 1300 independent local UK groups serving the needs of elderly people, assisted by well over 124 000 volunteers. The wide range of services provided includes advice and information, day care, visiting services, voluntary transport schemes, clubs and specialist services for physically and mentally frail elderly people.

Age Concern England
Bernard Sunley House
60 Pitcairn Road
Mitcham
Surrey CR4 3LL
Tel: 01-640 5431

Age Concern Scotland
33 Castle Street
Edinburgh EH2 3DN
Tel: 031-225 5000

Age Concern Wales
4th Floor
1 Cathedral Road
Cardiff CF1 9SD
Tel: 0222 371821/371566

**Age Concern
Northern Ireland**
6 Lower Crescent
Belfast BT7 1NR
Tel: 0232 245729

Introduction

This book is intended for practitioners from various disciplines who work with frail, vulnerable old people. It assumes that the reader will have a basic qualification of some kind but will not necessarily know a great deal about ageing, nor of the issues of policy and of service provision which arise in caring for such old people.

The main focus of the discussion is upon community care. Complex issues of care in hospitals for frail elderly people are not explored. The majority of hospital beds are occupied by elderly people and there is a need for the implications of this to be analysed. But that is another book! However, although about 95 per cent of elderly people live in their own homes, a minority need some form of residential care. Chapter 7 explores some of the complex problems involved in providing such care. Furthermore, the consideration of tending in Chapter 3 is of concern to all those, paid or unpaid, who care physically for old people. Increasingly, a sharp distinction between 'community' and 'residential' care is seen to be misleading and undesirable. We do not want old people's homes to be split off in this way; respite and short-term residential care and the use of homes for day care provision all emphasise a necessary relationship between the world outside and the world inside the institution.

There is much discussion at present about assessment. I have invited Michael Key to write a chapter on this topic because I believe that he has made an original and highly distinctive contribution to this most important subject and one which will be valued by professionals of all disciplines. In particular, what he has to say is in tune with the general theme of the book. It reinforces the attempt to understand old people, those he terms 'elders', at different levels and in different ways, in which the uniqueness of life experience is valued.

The way one views human behaviour and seeks to understand and explain it is profoundly affected by education and training. The approach in this book is, therefore, largely conditioned by my own educational experiences as a student, social worker and social work teacher. In particular, in my academic career, it has been important to bring together differing social and psychological perspectives in a manner which is helpful to prospective social workers. I am aware that these perspectives result in a different emphasis from those which others bring to work with old people. For example, doctors and nurses bring to it knowledge of biological and physiological systems and may have a detailed knowledge of the way these affect behaviour. Such considerations are not to be found in this book. That does not mean they are unimportant. On the contrary, the interface between health and social care is critical for the well-being of old people and this requires appreciation of, and respect for, the knowledge which all professions bring to their subject. However, many health professionals now find themselves working more and more outside the hospital, involved with others in making plans for social care in the community. It therefore seemed timely to reflect on these issues from what might be called a psychosocial perspective.

Social workers will be familiar with this way of looking at the world. However, it has become sadly apparent that many social work courses have not sufficiently explored these concepts and theories in work with old people. It is unlikely, therefore, that social workers will find the material in the book redundant.

The book has two central aims; firstly to demonstrate how interesting and how satisfying work with old people and their carers can be. Secondly, it is my hope and intention to claim for old people their proper place in the professional sun.

CHAPTER 1

Old age: Feelings, fears and attitudes

The purpose of this chapter is to open up for discussion some of the complex and ambivalent reactions which exist in us all towards old age and old people. In doing so it is inevitable that some of the negative aspects of ageing and our attitudes to it are stressed. This, of course, is only part of the story. We all know elderly people, including the very old, who relish life and are highly respected and loved by those around them. Indeed, even those who endure a great deal of suffering and loneliness will nonetheless claim that life still offers rich and satisfying experiences. In particular, there is a rapidly growing group of the 'young old', especially those with occupational pensions, who find themselves freed in retirement to develop interests and fulfilling activities unthought of in earlier years. They are not, however, the subject of this book. Vulnerable frail elderly people, usually the very old, are the group which give rise to most concern amongst carers, professional or personal. It is their position in society that this chapter addresses. Without greater honesty, we shall not combat effectively some of the extreme and ugly negativism which is widespread and which is epitomised by the derogatory phrases which Isaacs (1981) describes as 'defamatory' like 'old Crumble'.

A prerequisite in forming relationships with other people is empathy. We must have some conception of how other people feel. An imaginative response is at the heart of creative interaction. Nowadays, social value is ascribed to parents getting to know their children, in striking contrast to earlier centuries. Thus, intergenerational expectations are created; we say that we know what it is like to be a child; we have some understanding of the needs, joys and sorrows of childhood 'from the inside'. We are encouraged to make use of childhood experiences, rather than to discard them, especially in our interactions, such as play, with children.

Empathy is dependent in part on the ability to see similarities between the experiences of others and our own, even when these are not obvious. Barriers to empathy are created by some social structures and divisions, such as those of race, religion and class. It is also affected by our own capacity to bear the pain of others' experience. Everyone has to put limits on their emotional engagement with others – comprehensive engagement would be intolerable.

When we consider our reactions to old people, we must acknowledge that the barriers to empathy are considerable. By definition, we have not had the range of experiences which occur in old age, although we may well have some relevant personal knowledge upon which to draw. Are we to assume that old people's needs, joys and sorrows are the same as our own? At a very general and abstract level, this must be so – indeed, it is part of the prevailing ageism, which will be discussed later, that we often do not see old people as ordinary human beings with the same responses and reactions. However, when one becomes more detailed and specific, differences emerge, which it is not easy to envisage without personal experiences, either of one's own or of other old people. Take, for example, the near universal experience, in old age, of bereavement. Many of us in middle years of life have experienced the pain of such loss: few of us have experienced multiple losses, sometimes in quick succession, except in times of war; none of us have yet had to accept that those losses, of our own generation, signify the beginning of the end for us. What of joy? Is that too powerful a word for the positive experiences of old age? Or is that remark in itself ageist? Is joy, in contrast to sorrow, a more individual, idiosyncratic emotion about which generalisation is inappropriate? Is the fact that so few old people seem to express such strong positive feelings in itself significant of social, cultural and emotional deprivation? Is it a function of ageing or simply that the mode of communication may become more restrained and that the emotional experiences are as rich as ever? Simply asking these questions illustrates how little we know and understand and therefore how problematic an empathetic response may be.

The issue is further complicated by our attitudes to our own ageing. Can anyone put their hand on their heart and say that they are looking forward to very old age? Children cannot wait to be a year older ('I am five and three-quarters'), adolescents dream of marriage and careers, and people experiencing pressures of midlife may look forward to retirement and grand-parenthood. Would we believe someone who said they were viewing with enthusiasm the prospect of being 85? Some may be looking forward to the next life, others begin to take a pride in having reached advanced years, even in outliving others. But that is not the same as welcoming the prospect of that stage in life. Whether old people in societies which revere the wisdom and expertise of the very old would welcome advanced age, I do not know.

Thus, we do not know what it will feel like and we are not keen on knowing! We are fearful and anxious on our own behalf.

Expressions of apprehension are widespread in literature. One of the earliest and most vivid comes from the Bible:

> When thou wast young, thou girdest thyself and walkest whither thou wouldst; but when thou shalt be old, thou shalt stretch forth thy hands and another shall gird thee and carry thee whither thou wouldst not.
>
> (St John, 21. 18.)

Shakespeare's *King Lear* is the monumental tragedy of old age, in which total loss of self-esteem, based on royal status and self deception, leads to the disintegration of a proud man. Poets often express fear of ageing in terms of loss of physical beauty and sexual powers. A striking exception is to be found in Herbert's *The Flower*, one of the few poems to suggest that there can be growth, change and joy in old age.

> *Who would have thought my shrivelled heart*
> *Could have recovered greeness? It was gone*
> *Quite underground; as flowers depart to see their mother root,*
>   *when they have blown,*
> *Where they together*
> *All hard weather*
> *Dead to the world, keep house unknown.*
>
> *And now in age I bud again,*
> *After so many deaths I live and write;*
> *I once more smell the dew and rain, and relish versing.*

For younger people intimations of mortality may be unwelcome. Mysterious processes go on about this. I, and students to whom I have spoken, recall feelings of panic when facing the inevitability of our own death. Yet these feelings seem to diminish in intensity as one gets older. Presumably there are adaptive strategies to enable us to endure the unendurable. Very old people are often calm and commonsensical about their impending death in a way which can surprise and embarrass their younger visitors.

It has been suggested by McCullough (1981) that one of the problems in viewing old age constructively lies in the model of development customarily used by those who write about the life cycle. McCullough suggests that

> ... the paradigm of development as it is generally understood is not suited to explaining change in mature organisms. Futhermore, a constant emphasis on development in old age may be at variance with both our intellectual and our emotional response to decay and death.

He points out that

> ... initially gerontology itself was largely concerned with tracing decline in old age ...

and that present emphasis on development is an understandable reaction against this. McCullough argues that psychosocial changes in old people can be best understood by 'reference to social rather than developmental forces', that is to say, 'change in an individual may occur as a result of . . . interaction between internal and environmental factors'. Such a perspective enables one to view some of the more negative aspects of old age in contemporary society as being related to social factors in a given society. For example, McCullough cites the failure of Sibelius to compose for the last 20 years of his life as in part due to his discomfort at the rise of a genre of music with which he felt no affinity. In a more commonplace example, it does not take much imagination to see how old people may see their contribution to society as substantially diminished and their dependence increased, at a time when technological advances present an older generation with a succession of mysteries related to daily living.

Perhaps the most interesting point which arises from McCullough's article is that it needed to be said. Those who write about development in childhood, even those who stress predetermined norms, do not deny the impact of the environment on the child's social and emotional state. There is now quite an extensive sociological literature about old people, much of which draws attention to the various ways in which they are disadvantaged, even oppressed, through the creation of 'structured dependency'. Townsend (1981), for example, argues that

> Society creates the framework of institutions and rules with which general problems of the elderly emerge and indeed are manufactured.

He refers to

> . . . the committment of public expenditure which directly governs the services and benefits of older people in discussions about employment, wages and taxation, transport, urban planning and housing which have a powerful indirect effect on the situation and standard of living of the elderly.

However, such analysis has not been effectively related to the study of the ageing process from the point of view of the individual. What effect do these social forces have upon the functioning of old people, upon their morale, upon their enjoyment of life? To what extent are some of the so-called characteristics of ageing in fact social artefacts?

These questions must be addressed, even if they cannot be precisely answered; simply raising them has an effect on the way old people are viewed and the action which it is deemed appropriate to take. However, as with all discussion of the human condition, they have to be balanced with other considerations.

The first of these concerns the relation of the body to the mind and emotions. Some aspects of physical decline in old age are largely responsible for comparable decline in social functioning. Dementia is the most obvious, tragic and widespread example. Its biochemical causes are little understood but the effects of the disease in terms of organic deterioration are irrefutable and its effects on behaviour catastrophic. Whilst external social factors may be of some relevance to the management, even control, of the behaviour of those afflicted, the harsh fact is that external social influences play little part in its onset or progress. One may perhaps contrast this with the other common mental illness of old age, depression, in which loss, in many forms, from bereavement to loss of role and status, may reasonably be thought to play a part.

A secondary cautionary note about an approach to old age which stresses the significance of external social factors, arises from the existence of deeply ingrained antagonisms, even revulsion, towards old people. Jokes in literature about elderly cuckolds and misers are rife, some of which are uncomfortable for today's liberals, struggling to eradicate ageism from their consciousness. Such revulsion seems to be spiced with fear when old women, rather than men, are being talked about. Witches are more frightening then wizards, wolves lurk in grandmother's clothing. Margaret Drabble (1980) describes this well in *The Middle Ground*. Of a social worker, she writes:

> Evelyn . . . was actually frightened of the old and the frail. Ever since childhood, while talking to the very old, she had been frightened by visions of herself attacking, hitting, assaulting, knocking off their glasses. Evelyn, the mildest of women. These visions would appear, unsummoned, while she sipped cups of strong tea in clients' bedsitters. . . . Of course Evelyn knew that she would never assault an old person and that these horrid apparitions must be an image of her own fear of age and death, might even be some kind of safety valve. But they frightened her, nevertheless. . . . She was quite good with delinquent adolescents partly because she seemed to have some insight into the impulse that makes the young and the violent turn on the weak and the defenceless. . . . She was good also with parents who battered their babies, a less unusual talent. But she still, in her heart, grieved over her lack of easy contact with the frail. . . .

This seems more than a simple displacement of the fear and anxiety with which we contemplate our own old age. Are the old more likely to be invested with potential power, even supernatural? If so, why it is so often (though not universally) presented as evil? Such questions indicate how complex and deeply rooted are some of our negative attitudes to the aged. It may be that the best corrective to them arises from frequent interaction with a more benign reality. It has occurred to me to wonder what the previous experience has been of youngsters who savagely assault old people, whether they have ever been close to an old person. During a recent visit to an old people's home, the officer in charge told me of the efforts she had to make to prevent the local children from taunting and mocking the residents – often through the windows. One way was to seek to bring the children to meet the old people; yet, she told me, they were frightened to do so.

Thus, those who are committed to caring for and working with old people have first to face two facts. One is that strange and pervasive hostility to the aged, apparent from bygone days in myth and legend, survives in contemporary society. The second is that some elements of decline or decay are present in the ageing process and that these may on occasion substantially or totally affect social and emotional functioning. Work with old people which does not acknowledge this is based on a denial of reality, which does not provide a sound basis for our efforts. Furthermore, recognition of the significance of environmental factors upon the well-being of elderly people does not give us a magic wand; many of these factors are attributable to wider structural phenomena over which we and the elderly people have relatively little control. Of course, we can effect change and improvement for some and enjoy the sight of others who are well housed and well heeled. But the sheer numbers in relation to need can become overwhelming. Housing conditions and shortages, for example, are likely to be a major source of disadvantage and discomfort to millions of old people to the end of the century and beyond, and one on which individual workers, even managers, have relatively little impact. Even if one is not concerned with broader issues of social policy, one has at times a sense of being overwhelmed by the sheer extent of the work that needs to be done to support very old people and their carers, often reinforced by personal anxiety about one's own relatives.

The challenge, therefore, which confronts us is formidable. It is fashionable, nowadays, to write of 'isms' – racism, sexism and ageism, to name but three. (Disabledism has been tried, but it is an uncomfortable word.) 'Isms' describe negative attitudes towards a particular group of people. The reasons for these attitudes are bound up with complex and profound forces, as the preceding comments have indicated. Unfounded prejudice and stereotyping are characteristics of ageist attitudes. The process of stereotyping is part of the way in which we simplify the world. By picking on common characteristics of certain groups, we make it easier to sort people intellectually and there is nothing inherently unacceptable in it. It is rather like looking at people with a telescope rather than a microscope. At a distance people look more similar than different. Frequently, however, the generalisations are crude and misleading and antagonism is explicitly or implicitly present. Thus a process of distortion and exaggeration takes place because, at some level and for different reasons, we want to assert that 'they' (whoever 'they' may be) are not like us and are inferior in significant respects.

There has been more discussion of this phenomenon in relation to gender and race than age. Indeed, the fact that those lobbies are so much more vociferous than that for old people symbolises the problem which we have to confront: old people themselves are too accepting of the way they are viewed and described by others and others have been slow to take their part.

Ageism is pervasive and entrenched in our society. It finds various forms of expression. One of its most obvious, yet distressing, manifestations is the lack of discrimination between different ages covering 30 or more years. Indeed, to equate the age of retirement with old age is in itself arbitrary and problematic. If we were to shift the age of retirement down to 55 or up to 70, the people would still be the same! With reference to old people of over 75, who are here our main concern, there is a further aspect of ageist stereotyping which is prevalent and regrettable; that is, the tendency to make negative assumptions about the capacities of individual old people which are not based on a proper appraisal of their state. In attempting to combat ageist stereotyping, we have a problem. Unlike children, very old people do not have common 'norms of development' which can be used as quite a precise yardstick in the appraisals we all make of each other. (This lends weight to McCullough's argument, referred to earlier.) Old men and women over 75 vary greatly in physical and mental capacity which, of course, affects their social and emotional functioning. It is particularly important that those who work with and for elderly people keep a sense of perspective about this because, in their work, they will encounter a biased sample, those who need their help, many of whom do present serious problems.

Very large numbers of old people, especially women, live alone or with an elderly spouse and most manage their lives capably and competently. Younger people, abetted by the media, have a mode of comment about capable old people which seems to single them out as exceptional: 'Isn't she wonderful?'. Good stories are told and enjoyed; some old people are indeed exceptional, such as the man in his 70s who went parachuting recently, or the trenchant recollections of a man of 108 shown on television. But even this admiration can be a form of ageism if, by singling out the truly remarkable, we minimise the more mundane but no less significant achievements of so many very old people. Furthermore, some of those singled out for attention, judges, politicians and so on, occupying roles which attract attention and (sometimes!) respect, have clearly been endowed with exceptional qualities, of intellect and personality. In a sense, they do not help our cause.

Those who care for 'ordinary' old people learn much about the courage and competence which so many display; they discover that it is their ordinariness which is remarkable – their determination to carry on with the daily business of life, often in the face of considerable difficulties. Two examples, in particular, come to mind. Many old people have a severe degree of physical disability, of which rheumatism and arthritis top the lot for pain and discomfort. Perhaps everyone who works with such old people needs a period of physical disability (real or 'pretend') to see just what effort goes into the daily round and the strategies which are adopted the better to cope and to preserve independence. Yet this is commonplace. Commonplace, too, is loss of a spouse. Hundreds and thousands of men and women, especially women, live alone following such bereavement. Many were married from home and have not spent a night alone in the house all their lives. Many had, during marriage, distinct conjugal roles and were therefore quite unaccustomed to undertaking partners' household tasks. This kind of bereavement is not just about an emotional loss such as one experiences with the loss of a parent, however dear, with whom one does not live. It is about a crisis of identity (becoming a widow or widower), about facing aloneness, about developing new competencies, often at a time of life when physical strength and energy are diminished. Furthermore, loss of a spouse may occur at the same time as other bereavements.

The literature on bereavement, even that of Parkes (1986), which focuses on widows, has little to say about bereavement amongst very old people. There is no reference to old or elderly people in the index and the research cited does not single the very old out for comment. It is intriguing, however, to find, in the appendix, evidence from Parkes' study that the group of widows over the age of 65 showed a much smaller increase in sedative consumption after bereavement than those under 65 years old. Is this simply that older people use doctors less? Or are we seeing an indication that some inner processes of preparation for loss at this time of life have come into play? Are the reactions in the very old to bereavement the same as in younger people? Such are the questions which remain to be addressed. Perhaps the fact that those most frequently bereaved, the very old, have been the subject of so little research in this area, is in itself indicative of ageism amongst the professionals. Be that as it may, millions of old people make the necessary adjustment. They 'soldier on', and not infrequently find coping strength and skill which they did not know they had.

Although some people join the ranks of the old with relish and gloat over the advancing years ('I'm in my 80th year' – i.e. 79), others have commented on the incongruous feeling the idea of being old creates within them. Quite simply, they do not feel old, although they know with their minds they are. J.B. Priestley (1974) put it well:

> Being old is like playing a character role. Inside you're just the same. But you have a lot of stuff clamped on. Various ailments. They're no joke. . . . You're just the same inside. . . .

Many of the people we meet have lived alone since bereavement. Their loss is of companionship, quite simply, of someone to talk to.

> We needs words to keep us human. Being human is an accomplishment, like playing an instrument. It takes practice. . . . It is a skill we can forget.   (Ignatieff, 1984)

To combat ageism, therefore, we need knowledge and understanding of the effective adjustments which so many very old people make in the face of radically changed situations, physical, social and emotional. They are ultimately more instructive than stories of nonagenarians who scale Everest or even (enjoyable though they are) of Lord Denning's battles with the government from his seat in the House of Lords. We need above all, however, to approach all old people with the recognition that as individuals they are varied in their strengths and weaknesses, values and attitudes as the rest of us. (Admiration for the strong can turn into an implicit condemnation of the weak.) As individuals, too, they have the same human needs. To write this sounds platitudinous, yet to translate that understanding into daily practice is far more difficult than might at first appear. A particularly unpleasant and pervasive form of ageism is that which suggests that old people only require their basic physical needs to be satisfied, rather than a combination of physical, social, emotional and spiritual. I am ashamed to say that I have heard this said by social workers: 'all they really need is to be warm, comfortable and well fed'. Practices in some residential establishments illustrate this narrow conception of provision. Whilst physical infirmity may make physical care of great significance to the old person and mental infirmity may limit their capacity to give and receive other kinds of care, the efforts we make to relate to the whole person are critical if we are to avoid the stigmatising and depersonalising processes which insult the integrity of the old person.

Reference has already been made to the fact that most very old people are women. This means that gender-related attitudes affect them as well as those to do with ageing. Some of the primitive kind have already been alluded to, and are probably related to deep fears and fantasies associated with women. But these are filtered through social structures and affected by them so that the place of women in particular societies bears directly on their well-being in old age. Feminists have, until recently, paid scant attention to their older sisters but this is now being remedied. Some of the issues have been well described by the journalist, Barbara MacDonald (MacDonald and Rich, 1984), herself an elderly feminist.

> Ageism . . . is as old as the history of the family . . . men used family as a way of colonizing women as a class. Family was the original master servant model. . . . Familia is a male institution for controlling others.

There can be little doubt that attractiveness in women is more closely associated with sexuality and sexuality with youth, than is the case for men. It is socially acceptable for men to marry younger women, but not vice versa. It is commonplace to see middle-aged or elderly men as newscasters, but not yet women. Older women are sent daily signals that they must struggle to preserve their attractiveness. As Matthews (1979) puts it:

> That human bodies undergo biological changes as the years since birth accumulate cannot be denied. These changes are socially evaluated and are seen, for the most part, as negative: wrinkles are ugly while smooth skin is beautiful.

Of course, in a youth-orientated society, this applies to both men and women.

But few would deny that it bears more hardly on women. They must not be hairy in the wrong places but men can be bald!

Gender disadvantage is of course bound up with concepts of identity and role and may be more problematic for some newly retired men who have invested much in their world of work than for those women who have centred their existence in the home. But there are deep inequalities in the position of women which deserve analysis.

In this country, pioneering research by Finch and Groves (1983) drew attention to the extent to which social policies which place the main burden of family care on women affect their economic comfort and security in later life. As long as work in the home ('housework') is not formally remunerated, women reach old age without the same rights and entitlements as those in paid employment. This has been well illustrated in the present government's proposals for 'reform' of social security (DHSS, 1985/1986). SERPs (State Earnings Related Pension) will no longer be related to the best 20 years of earnings, a provision designed to take account of women's variable earnings pattern. Instead, some account (as yet unclear) will be taken of years out of the labour market. Furthermore, traditional dependence on a husband's earnings will be weakened (to an extent as yet unforeseeable) by higher divorce and remarriage rates.

For women whose self-esteem has been largely derived from being the centre of the home, there are a set of problems and issues to be resolved when they are required to take their place at the side of the family stage. As Matthews (1979) puts it, 'being An Old Mother in the unextended extended family'. Ubiquitous, often cruel, jokes about mothers-in-law underline these; how much pain they may give to some in the audience as they roll off the tongues of comedians.

There are further implications which arise from the mere fact that in contemporary society women live longer than men. There are so many of them around! Groups of women have in the past attracted ridicule ('hen parties') where male groups did not. This grows less but there is still some sense of unease; besides, many old women miss the company of men for social occasions. The structure of the social world of old people looks and feels abnormal. Staff of residential care establishments usually welcome more male residents and such men are 'a bit spoilt', both for their rarity value and perhaps because their domestic dependence is more acceptable.

Thus, whilst acknowledging that ageism creates problems for both men and women, it is important to pay special attention to the effect of gender on this and, in particular, to interaction of ageism and sexism.

In any consideration of old people in British contemporary society, the position of ethnic minority groups merits special attention. These issues have been excellently explored by Norman (1985) the title of whose book, *Triple Jeopardy*, describes a situation in which such old people are 'at risk because they are old, because of the physical conditions and hostility under which they have to live and because of services not accessible to them'. One might add a further definition of 'triple jeopardy' – they are old, mostly women and black, or in some way culturally distinct. Chapter 8 develops these points in more detail. In this introductory discussion, my concern has been to stress the need for empathy and the difficulties in achieving it in relation to old people. How much more difficult when that old person is of a different race or culture from one's own, has a lifetime of tradition and experience of which we know nothing and has been subjected to hostile experiences, whether the horror of the Holocaust or consistent denigration by virtue of skin colour?

Finally, we turn to a critical issue in any honest exploration of our attitudes towards old people, namely the value which our society ascribes to them. From what has been argued so far, it is apparent that there are powerful forces at work which tend to denigrate and diminish old people. Some of these are deeply rooted and irrational; they spring from fears about ageing and death and from the psychological need to distance ourselves from selected groups of people (homosexuals, blacks, etc.). However, we cannot leave it there. There are intransigent problems about the place of the very old in modern society. It has often been pointed out that in less developed societies, old people were seen as the repository of wisdom needed for daily living as well as for spiritual guidance. This contrasts with societies in which technological advance is so rapid that old people feel deskilled. One must be careful not to sentimentalise: more detailed anthropological studies would be needed to see how far this respect was diluted as frailty advanced or was ritually accorded, without substance. Yet there remains an important element of truth in the observation, 'another shall gird thee and carry thee whither thou wouldst not'. Recently, I went on a fishing trip in which the master was an old man, accompanied by a small boy. The roles of teacher and taught were clear, especially as he spoke gently to the boy showing him how to untangle a line – 'if you're mad with it, it will get mad back'. That illustrates nicely the interaction of practical and psychological guidance which characterises the best of apprenticeships. Such interaction is threatened when the pace of change is too fast or when the nature of that change is so radical as to transform the nature of the activity. The development of computers, in all their forms, is perhaps our most salient example. On a recent visit to a day centre, which served both younger disabled and old people, I was told that old people were envious and resentful when computer learning was introduced for the younger disabled people. They were also resistant to becoming involved, although it was not clear whether anyone had tried hard to encourage them. By contrast, the young ones were able to interest old people in the workings of microwave ovens; after cooking lessons from the young six or seven old people went out and bought them! What assumptions are we, and the old people themselves, making about their capacity to learn? How far is it affected by motivation, by a clear sense of purpose, as with the microwave ovens? But this is a digression. It must be acknowledged that very few very old people any longer feel that they have a significant contribution to make to the knowledge and skills which the young need to manage daily life. On the contrary, the roles are frequently reversed.

What then of emotional, even spiritual guidance? There are two contradictory images; an idealised one is of a benign, wise, peaceful old person, available to listen and perhaps to advise and to draw valuably upon life experience. Another, negative, image is of a draining, anxious old person, waiting for visits, immediately recounting the latest problems, perceived as trivial by the outsider, essentially self-absorbed.

The truth of the matter, of course, is that both exist, sometimes in the same person at different times. We have fallen into an ageist trap and attempted to generalise and to stereotype. To an extent, the use which the old can be to younger people is determined years earlier and is to do with the sort of people which they always were and their relationships with others. However, the patterns of modern living play a part. Old people who are not in frequent contact with younger people may lose confidence in their ability to give as well as to receive: Younger people, anxious to please, to give and, often, 'not to worry mother' may not realise the part which they play in creating a one-way traffic. Patterns of interaction are set up which do not encourage reciprocity.

When all allowance is made for such factors, it has to be said that as some people get older they do appear to show a marked increase in anxious self-absorption. To attribute this to the ageing process *per se* is as foolish as it is to describe physical disease as 'your age, my dear'. It should lead us to reflect further on the messages which such behaviour is intended to convey. Depression in old age is common and is often marked by anxiety. Loneliness and isolation are widespread as are pain and discomfort. Many old people spend long hours alone and many are increasingly fearful (rightly or wrongly) of violence in the street or at home. Thus, whilst not discounting the possibility of a long-standing personality trait, the appeal for imaginative empathy with which this chapter began is also its ending. 'How would I feel in these circumstances?' is not a bad beginning, although it cannot be an ending.

CHAPTER 2

The emotional and social significance of dependence in old age

The words 'dependent' and 'independent' are frequently used with reference to elderly people. They are used in a wide variety of ways, covering many different aspects of human existence, and there are often unexplored value judgements inherent in them. This chapter seeks to explore these matters in some depth, for they are critical to the understanding of elderly people.

Reference has earlier been made to the now extensive literature on the 'structured dependence' of the elderly, to which, in this country, Townsend (1981) and Walker (1981) have been significant contributors. The pervasive consequences of 'structured dependency' have been excellently drawn together by Phillipson and Walker (1986) who have edited a book which explores the policy implications of the phenomenon. They consider, *inter alia*, the position of old people in regard to health and housing provision. Townsend's thesis is that in four main areas, 'the dependency of the elderly in the twentieth century is being manufactured socially'. These are:

> the imposition and acceptance of earlier retirement; the legitimation of low income; the denial of rights to self determination in institutions; and the construction of community services for recipients assumed to be predominantly passive.

Townsend asserts that the extent of that dependence is unnecessary and that 'the process can . . . be revised or least modified'.

Walker (1981) draws particular attention to poverty in old age, arguing that it is 'primarily a function of low economic and social status prior to retirement and the depressed social status of the retired, and, secondly of the relatively low level of state benefits'. He claims that widespread poverty amongst elderly people has been relatively ignored by academics and politicians, although it has resulted in the 'social creation of dependent status'.

A consequence of these processes, as Walker puts it, has been 'periodic expressions of alarm at the "burden" of dependency' which old people create for the rest of us. (Children, the other main economically dependent group, are not usually referred to as burdens.) This unattractive and socially divisive reaction has been reinforced by government publications (DHSS, 1985/86) on the 'reform' of social security in which the potential burden on the tax payer of pension provision was put forward as a primary reason for the changes.

In Britain, in the last ten years, the picture is confused. There is greater awareness amongst those who work with and for the elderly of the ways in which we manufacture social and economic dependency. At the level of the individual, efforts have been made to promote practices in residential and, to a lesser extent, in community care which will enhance old people's rights to greater control over their own lives. The code of practice *Home Life* (1984), commissioned by the government and produced by the Centre for Policy on Ageing, is a contemporary example of this. It is widely used as a kind of yardstick for good practice. Yet most would agree that, whilst good intentions flourish, we have barely begun a process to which sensitising staff is the key. Furthermore, there can be little doubt that the sudden and huge growth in private residential care and nursing homes raises new problems, since there can be so little detailed control of the quality of care.

There are also important questions to be asked about the reasons for admission to residential care in the first place, for that in itself is an aspect of dependency. Townsend's earlier work (1961) showed a high proportion of residents lacked orthodox family support, for example, had not been married. More recently (1981) he has raised the question of the process by which people are admitted, for instance through homelessness following hospitalisation. Thus, factors largely outside the control of the old person can create a dependency upon institutional care. We are now faced with a wave of admissions to private residential care. The reasons for it remain to be fully understood but it will certainly reopen the debate about this aspect of dependency – chosen or enforced?

When we turn to the 'macro' issues which Townsend and Walker address, the picture is gloomy. Rising unemployment gives no hope of raising the age of retirement. Rightly or wrongly, such a move would be seen as 'taking jobs from younger people'. Not everyone, however, accepts the desirability or feasibility of a longer working life. Some believe that we should be looking at all ages to fulfilling activity which is not wholly employment based, but make more constructive use of leisure. That, of course, is bound up with the issue of income maintenance. Retirement in poverty may offer little scope for creative use of leisure. The publication *Manifesto for Old Age* by Bornat *et al.* (1985), serves only to highlight the yawning gulf between aspiration and reality, in a range of critical areas of social policy for older people, such as income maintenance, housing and education. On the first of these, as has already been indicated, recent legislation and policies have actually been detrimental to the interests of many old people. Their entitlement under the State Earnings Related Pensions Scheme (SERPs) will be curtailed, though public pressure compelled the government to give up its intention to discard the scheme in favour of private pensions. Equally – perhaps more seriously – the relative value of the basic pension has been falling because it has been related to prices, not incomes, so that unless steps are taken, by the year 2025 the value of the basic pension as a proportion of gross earnings could have fallen by half.

The financial consequences of the past and present policies have resulted in 'two worlds' of old people: those with the security of good occupational pensions, to whom a wide range of attractive retirement options are open; and those whose dependence on means-tested supplements to their basic pensions necessitates dependence of a personal and immediate kind upon the state, and whose quality of life is restricted by their financial circumstances. In this last group, black elderly people are over-represented because they have often not worked in this country long enough to accumulate full pension entitlement. For obvious reasons, financial security at a level which permits old people to join in the activities which are part of everyday society is a foundation on which much else rests. It is a necessary, but not always sufficient, condition for well-being and for the reduction of one aspect of dependency in old age.

The analysis of the factors leading to structured dependency in old age is a powerful one, bound up with economic policies, which are determined, as always, by values, and essentially moral choices about priorities. Some government statements have come perilously close to saying 'we cannot afford old people' and those who care for old people must not be diverted from a moral stand by economic filibustering. But, as Townsend suggests, structured dependence is not only about macro-economic and social issues. It concerns how we design and provide services, and therefore it is within our power as individual workers to effect some improvements.

In a sense, much modern human life is about structured dependency. The pervasive and complex systems of economic dependency in developed countries ensure that we are interdependent in innumerable critical ways and may readily be made to feel powerless. Whilst things go smoothly, much of this goes without attention, but wars, strikes and other disruptions periodically jolt us. Reactions are sometimes excessive and irrational, suggesting that we depend more for our self-confidence on such reliable systems than we may care to realise. A bread strike offers a good example. Long queues for that symbolic food, the staff of life, will immediately materialise, despite the ready availability of many alternatives.

For very old people, whose security and confidence in these matters may revolve around a relatively small number of tried and tested commodities and services, their withdrawal may be experienced as particularly threatening.

High on the list of their priorities will be, of course, heating. Fears and anxieties surrounding the provision of adequate warmth may be a rational response to the external situation, or, on occasion, excessive.

We are also all dependent on external systems for the maintenance of our dwellings and essential equipment. For very old people, this poses particular problems. The conventional notion of a simple customer transaction conceals a host of difficulties, bound up with the financial power of the old customer, the status of old people more generally, the limited capacity which many have, especially women alone, to do their own repairs, the shortages of special services in given areas, and so on. For many in local authority or privately rented accommodation, the sense of frustration and powerlessness can be overwhelming. Here money in your pocket (or savings bank) is irrelevant.

All this is, of course, true for others beside old people, and it is no part of the argument to categorise old people so separately as to further stigmatise them. But, in the nature of things, old people spend much more time indoors. Not surprisingly, the defects in dwellings or the equipment on which they depend loom large. They suffer more, as a result, both physically and emotionally – the dripping tap drips on the emotions, like Chinese torture. Those who work with elderly people may have noticed that these (sometimes apparently trivial) domestic problems create anger and despair when they cannot be resolved. They bring home dependency – in a painful way. They may reawaken memories of happier times – 'my husband would have done that in five minutes'. This present dependence on others for the correction of minor matters may trigger more profound resentment in old people about the degree and nature of the dependence in which old age has placed them.

At a more intimate and personal level, the balance between independence and dependence raises fascinating issues which have as yet been little explored in relation to old age. Since, throughout our lives, we seek a balance which is comfortable for us, it will be no different for old people but may be much more difficult to achieve. This balance changes throughout the life cycle. Just as infants are totally dependent for physical and emotional care on parent figures, so there are some very old people, and others who are terminally ill, for whom this total care is now necessary. It is generally provided by relatives or by staff in hospitals or nursing homes. When this care of old people is short-lived, the inevitable prelude to death, it is accepted as natural. This is, after all, the meaning of the phrase 'life cycle'. How we see it is affected by our culture and religious faith. That final dependence may be experienced as distressing or peaceful, but it is not socially problematic.

Increasingly, however, the phase of such near total dependence is protracted by severe physical or mental infirmity, such as that caused by a stroke or dementia. In such a phase, there may be little interpersonal gratification for those who care and are cared for except at the level of the meeting and satisfaction of basic human needs, unless there is a kind of 'love bank' in the carer from earlier days. Even when the carer is a relative, when dementia is the disease carers may feel as if the old person has in a sense already died and left them so that 'this is not the mother I used to know'. Increased life expectancy has brought with it a major burden (the word is here used advisedly) and responsibility in the care of those in an advanced state of mental and physical decline.

Long before that stage is reached, however, questions about dependence trouble and puzzle many old people and those who care for them. There are many different facets. One concerns the domains of independence which are most cherished by a particular person. Most of us seek to preserve independence in matters in which the bodily functions of urinating and excreting are concerned. To relinquish autonomy in that area will be experienced as unwelcome by nearly everyone who is mentally normal, which is hardly surprising given the importance ascribed to the achievement of continence in childhood. For that reason alone, everyone who works with very old people needs to be aware of the emotional and social impact of incontinence. Williamson (1981) puts it well in relation to urinary incontinence. How much more so for faecal incontinence!

> The onset of bladder dysfunction . . . leads to considerable distress and embarrassment. The old lady who dare not allow herself to be more than a few yards from the toilet or the old man whose underclothes are frequently wet with urine, may often react by limitation of social life and consequent days of isolation and low morale. . . .

A consequence of this may be to increase the dependence of the old people on others because they will need their help to get to the toilet and use it. Those of us who make our own way there have little conception of the anxiety this may induce, unless, perhaps, we have waited for bedpans in hospital. Sadly, this vulnerability may be used in power games between staff and residents in homes, or between residents. I have heard of old women who forbid others in their lounge to go to the toilet when they appear to do so too frequently.

The significance of these matters for the well-being of individual old people is now much more widely recognised, witnessed by the increasing use of continence advisors, who can do much to prevent and ameliorate the problem. Yet they have only touched the tip of the iceberg, especially with respect to old people in their own homes or private care. If we are right in regarding it as the single most important area in which independence is prized and which also causes major distress for carers, it seems clear that it should be a priority in health and social services provision.

It is interesting that this may be the only area in which dependence is almost universally feared and resented. Even other intimate bodily functions, such as bathing, do not necessarily raise such feeling. It is here that the endless varied reactions of individuals make the task of caring for old people so fascinating and so complex. For our attitudes towards specified aspects of dependence and independence are an amalgam of past experiences, personality traits and present circumstances.

Of past experiences we can only speculate. It seems obvious that they are relevant but how precisely they interact with present behaviour is unclear. Much dependence in old age has a major physical component; many old people need help in walking, bathing, feedings, dressing and so on. All these activities are the stuff of childhood and mastery of the tasks involved are minor landmarks. Of what is our adult self-esteem composed? How important is physical competence, as compared, for example, with intellectual or social competence? What enables us to give up physical areas of independence 'gracefully'? Perhaps, though regrettably, they are not seen as a central core of independence which may reside elsewhere – 'in my head or in my dreams'. Perhaps such physical dependence is not unwelcome, recalling memories of childhood which are tender and warm. On a recent visit to a day centre, where a large number of old people had regular baths, I was told that bath time was a time for confidences and chats. Numerous sponge bags hung on pegs, some with rubber ducks poking out! In such intimate matters, one would expect that the feelings of the old person about their body and the extent to which 'family frankness' has been part of earlier experience would also play a part. (Sexual intimacy does not necessarily mean that old people have been frank about their bodies.)

All kinds of life experiences go into the making of an old person who enjoys this and does not enjoy that. Acceptance, dependence or rejection will therefore be inextricably tied in with the preservation of areas of activity which have given self-esteem, which are associated with a particular role function, which confirm the old person as the sort of person he or she wants to be. Conversely, it may not be hard to relinquish certain roles and tasks which were never experienced as rewarding. It is not uncommon to hear of old women who are cross when asked to perform domestic tasks in residential care! The phrase 'I've been doing it all my life' may mean 'in this role I am confident and feel fulfilled'. It may mean 'this is a role which was ascribed to me as a woman and which I resented'.

Those who work with old people might consider compiling a list of regular tasks or activities and, as part of planned intervention, finding out what are most and least precious areas of independence to old people – choosing clothes, managing money, cleaning the kitchen, going shopping and so on. For it has to be remembered that very old people get very tired and need to be selective about activity. It is sad when the options are closed off because those who support do not know what is of most significance.

The balance of dependence and independence in precious long-standing relationships, usually husband and wife, sometimes (and importantly) between siblings or parents and children, plays a part in current behaviour. Patterns get established over time which colour present behaviour. Sometimes it is manifested in an exaggeration of previous dependency when problems arise; sometimes, with strangers, excessive expectations of and need for support arise from these earlier relationships ('My husband waited on me hand

and foot.') However, we are in a shadowy area unless we have some second-ary verification of how those relationships worked. Idealisation of past rela-tionships may reflect unsatisfied longings; what is reported may be how old people would like it to have been. Nor should we ever underestimate the capacity of old people to alter life-long patterns of interaction when need arises. This is particularly well illustrated in the case of old men who devote themselves to providing near total care for ailing wives, many having gone through marriage with little domestic involvement. If there is one lesson to emerge from consideration of the changing balance of dependence and inde-pendence in old age, it is the flexibility and adaptability for which old people are given so little credit.

The kind of situations in which old people find themselves is another salient factor in considering dependence and independence. Implicit in what has already been said is the inescapable fact that many old people have, by reason of physical frailty, a degree of enforced dependence which is unwelcome. If to that we add both the structured dependency which was earlier described, in which social policies and practices discriminate against them in matters crucial to their well-being (such as housing, income and transport), and the personal indignities of physical and social dependence, we must surely put at the top of our agenda for care a determination to assess realistically, yet sensitively, what is the best balance that can be achieved in the present circumstances of that old person. Those circumstances are not, however, static. In matters of this kind we are often considering a span of 15–20 years from the time when it is first apparent that an old person cannot 'carry on as before' to the time of death. Nor is this necessarily a model of steady decline. On the contrary, there are often years on an even plateau, and periods of greater dependence, after bereavement for example, which are subsequently reversed. For those, usually relatives, who are involved in this lengthy period, and who are often concerned and loving, and for the old person themselves, more general help and advice on some of the problems associated with growing more frail would be of value in easing the transition and preventing precipitate actions (such as selling the house), which will afterwards be regretted.

For those who become involved at a stage when there is a high degree of frailty, there are many sensitive decisions in daily caring which can slow down or halt the progress of dependence. Sadly, work like this is critically affected by staffing levels, whether in institutional or community care. There is no doubt that sustaining and fostering independence takes time – a scarce resource. Doing 'for' rather than 'with' people usually takes longer.

In any discussion of dependence and independence, the balance of power between individuals has to be taken into account. Obviously, frail elderly people are physically less powerful than those who look after them and in certain circumstances this may have a significant effect on their state of mind. In particular, rough handling by 'carers' – whether relatives, care staff or even ambulance men – may engender considerable anxiety. However, power is about more than physical strength. Literature is replete with tales of the power which old people have exercised over property and the way this has been used in intergenerational interactions. More complex still is emotional power, for example, the kind of interaction which we describe as 'emotional black-mail', in which one party is made to feel guilty at failing to meet the perceived needs of the elderly person. Indeed, it may be that on occasion physical ill-treatment is a consequence of the tension this sort of situation produces.

This illustrates a central concern of this book, that we should at all times view old people as playing a part in the drama of life, not as passive onlookers. The logical consequence of this is that they will on occasion play unattractive parts!

Because we are more dependent and more vulnerable in later years, there has rightly been concern about what may be termed 'old age abuse' and the subject merits some detailed discussion here. The research literature, mostly emerging from the USA, has many parallels with earlier writing on the subject of child abuse. There are the same problems in estimating incidence, in defining the phenomena and in defining the characteristics of the abuser or the situations which give rise to abuse.

There seems little point in wasting research time on the incidence of old age abuse; as with child abuse, it can lead to a kind of spurious precision, in which figures are cited which will not bear scrutiny for three main reasons. Firstly, unless and until definitions are agreed, we may be attempting to compare the incidence of different phenomena. Secondly, the estimates are based on *reported* abuse, which is dependent on the highly variable practices of agencies and practitioners. Thirdly, by its very nature, abuse is likely to be 'hidden' and difficult to discover (except in its grossest forms), with the abused person, as well as the abuser, having a stake in keeping it secret. However, what is needed on the part of practitioners is a raised level of awareness of the problem and a willingness to entertain the possibility that it exists. In this we have much to learn from child abuse. One of the most striking and curious aspects of the social history of child abuse is the way in which it was denied and ignored by the professionals, notably doctors. Physical abuse was 'discovered' in the 1960s. It is now almost impossible to imagine how doctors did not diagnose it before. We are now confronting a similar situation with regard to child sexual abuse. The flood of referrals now reaching health and social services does not, of course, mean that a new evil is stalking the land. It means that public awareness has been raised and that professionals are (more or less) willing to entertain the possibility of its occurrence. Such social pro-cesses make us aware how immensely powerful are the mechanisms of denial, the psychological capacity to shut our eyes and ears to matters which are too painful to be contemplated and which create for practitioners ethical and professional dilemmas which are hard to resolve. It seems clear that we face a similar (though not identical) situation with regard to old age abuse. It remains to be seen whether we can learn by analogy. Meanwhile, rather than trading figures, the need is for openness to the idea. It should come as no surprise that, in a society with increasing numbers of very old people, proportionately and absolutely, a substantial proportion of whom have a serious degree of mental infirmity, a significant number will suffer abuse.

As with child abuse, defining old age abuse is a problem for those who wish to undertake research. There are various suggested categories: direct physical or sexual abuse; physical neglect; psychological abuse, such as verbal threats; material abuse, such as theft of money; and violation of rights, such as forcing an old person into a home against their will (Sengstock and Liang, 1982). Obviously, some or even all of these may be present in one case. Psychological abuse probably poses the greatest difficulty in trying to decide what is beyond the bounds of socially acceptable behaviour towards an old person. Important as it is to recognise that the notion of abuse has wider connotations than the physical, not much purpose seems to be served by struggling to define more precisely such elusive matters as emotional interactions. Rather, it seems preferable that, in making a general assessment of the quality of life of a particular old person, some attempt be made to examine the negative and positive aspects of the relationships which they presently experience.

Research and writing on this subject has concentrated almost exclusively on abuse by family members and most of it occurs in the domestic setting. Yet it is self-evident that it may occur in other situations, most particularly in institutional care. Where such establishments are subject to careful 'quality control', one would hope not to find physical abuse or neglect in their grosser forms. Yet it should never be forgotten that some of the disquiet felt about institutional care (more fully discussed in Chapter 7) has arisen from the 'scandals' of chronic wards in hospitals, in which long-term patients were, on occasion, subjected to degrading treatment. At the present time, there are grounds for similar concern about both the public and the private sector. It is clear that mechanisms for quality control are not adequate.

Why then are old people abused by those who look after them? It is highly unlikely that research will do more than elaborate and refine matters upon which one may reasonably speculate from experience, from theories of behaviour generally, and from knowledge available from other areas, such as child abuse, or particular to ageing.

Firstly we must link the problem to attitudes to old people generally. We have earlier discussed the prevalence of ageism. Inherent in such attitudes is denigration of old people. There is a terrifying slippery slope in the process, by which old people come to be regarded as less than fully human and are therefore not treated as persons deserving equal respect. This may be exacerbated by their mental frailty or by their neglected appearance (a vicious circle in this context) or by sensory deficits such as deafness.

Secondly, in family abuse, the history of the relationships may be of great significance in current abuse. On occasions, current behaviour is simply a repetition of long-standing family patterns, as for example when there has been marital conflict expressed in physical violence or where a mentally ill son or daughter has had periodic outbursts of physical aggression. In such cases, the physical frailty of the old person may be the only element in the situation which has changed.

Whether or not there has been any history of violence, the association between the past and the present is bound to be significant in understanding present abuse within the family. It is in this area that more clinical research might most profitably be done, for these are complex psychological phenomena about which we have little certainty. For example, it has been suggested that sons or daughters may resent a situation in which they find themselves forced to be 'in charge' of a formerly dominant parent. Or there may be an element of retaliation for past suffering.

Thirdly, both in families and institutions, sadism is occasionally encountered. Sadistic people derive perverse pleasure from the suffering of others and may seek out situations in which they can inflict this. Again, it has been suggested that this is associated with past experiences of violence on the part of the abuser. Although it is important to seek to understand the roots of sadism if one is to help the person to change, those who care for elderly people will be primarily concerned to protect them. In institutional care there should be no place for such people. When the old person is in a family, complex and as yet unresolved issues are raised concerning the introduction of legal powers which would enable the abused person to be removed. (We return to these matters at the end of this chapter.)

Acknowledging that ageism, family discord and psychopathology all play their part in abuse, it is situational stress which is probably the most significant factor in those many episodes which fall short of systematic and gross abuse but which nevertheless cause great distress and suffering. It is also the factor most likely to be remediable by practitioners.

In the succeeding chapters, the role of carers, paid and unpaid, is explored at considerable length. Increased understanding of the burdens which they carry should lead us to greater awareness of the strain under which they are so often put. There are two matters which merit particular attention in relation to abuse. One concerns their reaction to 'mess'. The physical care of frail old people necessarily involves much attention to food and to toileting. Old people, perhaps mentally infirm, who spit out food when it is given, or who lose the capacity to eat tidily and whose bowel and bladder functioning is impaired, may rouse deep feelings of revulsion in carers, of which they were quite unaware until confronted with the behaviour. This is particularly likely to provoke hostility when it is believed that there is an element of wilfulness in the old person's responses. For example, it is not uncommon to hear that the carer 'cracked' when a parent is incontinent immediately after leaving the toilet. It is interesting to contrast this with similar descriptions in child abuse in which, for example, a baby is punished for being dirty, the expectations of the parent being quite unrealistic. The extent to which particular old people can control their behaviour and to which certain actions are an expression of hostility is problematic. But if it is experienced as hostile, it may provoke the carer into actions which are atypical and frequently followed by remorse and guilt. People vary greatly in their tolerance of 'mess', which no doubt is rooted in their own personality and childhood experiences.

A second element in much situational stress arises in the care of those suffering from severe dementia. Such old people customarily exhibit behaviour which is extraordinarily difficult to tolerate and which raises a high level of anxiety. Carers are ever conscious of danger and often of restless and agitated behaviour which pervades the household. Small wonder then, that restraint on occasion gives way to abuse, especially given the failure of our formal systems to offer adequate support.

Whilst these problems arise acutely for family carers, who are so often grievously isolated socially, they are also salient to care staff in institutions, especially when staffing levels are inadequate. Unacceptable practices which have an abusive component, such as tying old people to commodes, are much more likely to arise when there are insufficient numbers of staff to complete the ascribed tasks.

Situational stress, however, is not only related to the actions or behaviour of the person being cared for. It is bound up with the family as a whole. An approach to family functioning which emphasises the interactions of each upon the other and their cumulative impact is essential if we are to understand adequately the position of an old person at a given time. This applies not only to the small number of the very old who live in three-generational households, although that throws up some particular issues and problems, it is equally relevant when there are triangular interactions, such as husband, wife and old person, or to situations when the old person lives alone but is closely supported by kin. It has further been suggested by Sengstock and Liang (1982) that abuse frequently occurs at times when other problems, both practical and emotional and not specifically connected with the old person, are occuring in the family. It would not be surprising to find that material and social deprivation play a part in increasing stress and propensity to abuse, especially when associated with isolation.

In making these comments, one begins to ask, 'why is it necessary that they be made?'. Is it not all blindingly obvious? There is nothing here that a good social worker with families, for example, would not know about. Yet over and over again, one finds that the application to problems in old age has to be made, that prevailing attitudes have discouraged appropriate and sensitive appraisal of the intergenerational or marital dynamics, and of the emotional reactions of carers, which can lead to abuse.

Reference was made earlier to financial abuse. There are matters here which are of great social concern and which are excellently discussed by Greengross (1986), in *The Law and Vulnerable Elderly People*. These concern the confused and inadequate systems which at present exist to protect old people's money and property. They cannot be adequately explored here, but practitioners are urged to read Greengross' book and to consider the position of old people with whom they work.

Practitioners concerned about suspected or actual abuse of old people will often be perplexed as to the best course of action. Where carers admit that abuse has occurred, or are fearful that it may, the worker may have the opportunity to work with the carer (and where possible, the old person) on a future strategy. This may be focused on support to relieve stress, the modification of certain behaviour or interactions, or the need for the parties to separate. The last is usually to be regretted but there have been occasions when long-standing marital unhappiness was resolved by admission to residential care in the last years. More often, of course, separation involves a younger carer giving up the role, about which there is often profound ambivalence. The manner in which people are helped with those confused and painful feelings may have considerable significance for their future mental health.

There will be other situations in which abuse is not admitted. Where the evidence seems incontrovertible, it may sometimes be desirable to confront the persons concerned, even to the point of suggesting that a referral to the police might be made. Some social workers have found that such directness produced an admission which enabled some honest work to take place and help to be offered. But that is clearly a radical step, only likely to be taken when very serious abuse is involved.

A central problem in working with such cases concerns the position of the old person in question, who has been abused. Their wishes and feelings are, or should be, of primary concern. They are adults, not children, which places practitioners in a different relationship to them, in which their rights to determine their own lives are accepted, unless they are 'incompetent' to do so. It is common for old people to play down the extent of the abuse and it is not easy to gauge how far their reluctance to discuss alternative care is due to fear of the unknown rather than acceptance of the situation. Furthermore, decisions as to 'incompetence' are highly complex. On the one hand, it may well be felt that an old person's wish to stay with a carer should be respected unless their mental state is so gravely impaired that they literally do not know what they are doing. On the other hand, fear of the unknown, shame at admitting that relatives have harmed them, and fear of retribution may create a kind of mental and emotional paralysis which is not the same as a positive wish to stay at home.

The present legal position does not cater adequately for such contingencies, as Greengross (1986) has cogently pointed out. As things stand, a dilemma of this kind can only be resolved through the use of cumbersome legal machinery which is not appropriate to the situation. There are two relevant statutes. One, Section 47 of the National Assistance Act 1948, allows for the forcible removal from their own homes of elderly people who are not mentally ill. This provision has been the subject of wide-ranging criticism (Norman, 1980; Greengross, 1986). It is now generally applied to those who have neglected themselves over a long period of time or when a person has become seriously ill but is refusing hospital admission. Although the wording of the Act suggests that it could be used in cases of abuse, it seems that there is such a general sense of unease about the law as it stands that some new and especially designed statute will be necessary for effective provision.

The second relevant statute concerns guardianship under the Mental Health Act 1983. The person (of any age) must suffer from a mental disorder as defined in the Act and enforced guardianship must be necessary for the welfare of the patient or the protection of others. A guardian must be either a local social services department or a person accepted by them. Such orders last initially for six months but this can be extended. In cases of abuse, two problems may arise. Firstly, the old person must be clinically diagnosed as mentally ill. Secondly, if the nearest relative objects an order can only be made by application to the county court, which would complicate and delay the process.

If an offence has been committed against the person, the police can of course bring charges and, under certain conditions, make an arrest. However, the granting of bail is the most likely outcome. This means that the old people would be left with the abusers unless they wanted to go into care or unless they were themselves mentally impaired. In the latter case, they could be made the subject of a Mental Health Order, but there is little precedent for so doing. It seems clear that, with careful safeguards, we need some legal machinery, similar to the provision of Place of Safety Orders for children, by which an old person could be received into residential care for their own protection, at least for a limited period of time, which would afford a breathing space for all concerned and enable a proper assessment to be made of the situation – including the wishes of the old person once they were out of the violent or neglectful environment. Greengross (1986) has suggested that an 'intervention order' might be granted by a magistrate in these circumstances. She points out that at present local authorities have no duty to investigate alleged abuse, as in child abuse, and suggests this should be remedied. In carrying out its duty to consider and assess the needs of a vulnerable elderly person, the local authority should:

1. consider and take into account the wishes expressed by the elderly person and assess that person's needs;
2. assess the need of the carer for support and help in the tasks being carried out on behalf of the vulnerable elderly person and in providing care;
3. review the needs of the elderly person and/or the carer at intervals of not more than twelve months, until or unless the review considers this to be unnecessary;

4. consider whether it would be appropriate to appoint an inde-
    pendent person to be a 'visitor'.

(Greengross, 1986)

If such an investigation led to the decision to seek the removal of an old person
from their home, an intervention order could be applied for, with emergency
provisions as necessary.

While the need to protect old people and their carers from unwarrantable
intrusion is of great importance, it would seem that there is a strong case for
new legal provisions to afford better mechanisms for protecting old, abused
people, in the community and in residential care. It is to be hoped that we will
not need a scandal to bring it about.

Physical abuse is not known to be extensive and it may be felt that it has
been excessively discussed in the context of 'dependence and independence'.
I believe, however, that the emphasis is justified because it has received so
little systematic attention in the British literature. Age Concern's useful literature review (Cloke, 1983) showed how little we really know. In Britain, Eastman (1984), a social worker, is one of the few who have sought to draw
attention to abuse of old people. Unfortunately, his concern about the issue
does not seem to be adequately conceptualised nor related to more general
issues concerning the strains on family life. To separate consideration of old
age abuse from the range of powerful emotions, positive and negative, which
are present in those who depend and those who care, and which affect all
interactions, is both limiting and stigmatising. The dangers of such an
approach have been seen in comparable work with children and families.
That is not to say, however, that we should collude in a denial of the phenomenon. Hence the attention that it has been given here.

Will we see scandals, even inquiries, in future concerning old age abuse, as
we have seen them with children? Sadly, there must be some cause for them.
Does the general public care less about the plight of some old people than it
does about children? Will greater professional awareness raise public consciousness? These are matters on which we must ponder.

In concluding this chapter, I return to the more general theme of the
balance in the last years of life between dependence and independence. It will
be apparent from the earlier discussion that a simple assertion about helping
old people maintain their independence does not do justice to the subtleties of
achieving a balance between independence and dependence which is acceptable or tolerable to the old people concerned. This is not to disparage in any
way the commitment of health workers to physical rehabilitation which will
sustain or restore people's physical independence, especially following illness
or accident. However, it is well known that the motivation of the person
concerned is an important ingredient in successful independence. If that
motivation appears to be weak or there is marked ambivalence, it is worth
reflecting upon what the old person wants to be able to do! Thus, the objective

of caring work should be twofold. Firstly, it is to seek to preserve, even to restore, areas of autonomous functioning which are important to the integrity and self-esteem of a particular old person. Secondly, it is to ensure that, so far as possible, appropriate dependence is enjoyed, and occurs in a climate of warmth and affection. If that has resonances of childhood which the very old, whose full circle is nearly complete, find agreeable, so be it. That is not patronising, it is loving.

CHAPTER 3

Care in the community I: The social context

This topic has been extensively discussed. It has been rhetorically espoused by politicians and sceptically analysed by academics. It is now commonplace to draw a distinction between care *in* and care *by* the community. The former term simply describes the situation in which people live outside institutions; the latter points to the support which such people may receive from others. For the old people who are the subject of this book, some care *by* the community is essential if they are to stay *in* it. It is most important for those who develop services for old people to consider the complexities and variations of the social structures which we describe with words like 'community', 'neighbourhood' and 'networks' – all overworked and imprecise terms as presently used by many professionals.

The focus of this discussion is upon old people living in private households. (Whether old people living in residential homes can be said to be living in the community is a separate issue, some aspects of which are considered in Chapter 7.) The importance of the support which is offered to old people in such private households cannot be overestimated. The 1981 census showed that nearly 97 per cent of people of pensionable age were thus accommodated; while the recent dramatic growth of private residential care may increase the proportion in institutional care, the fact remains that they will remain a minute fraction of the elderly population. We should further note the dramatic increase, postwar, in numbers of old people living alone. The 1961 census found 18.9 per cent of all elderly persons living alone. By 1981, this had risen to almost one third (29.9 per cent), that is 2¾ million (Family Policy Studies Centre, 1984). Many more women over 85 live alone – 53 per cent in 1980 (OPCS, 1980). The trend continues upward.

A further 44 per cent of all elderly people live only with a spouse and, as we saw in the last chapter, only about 14 per cent are living with others – 'non-spouses'. Thus, although until recently the position of those who are tended by and 'tend' old people in the same household has been too little discussed and merits more sensitive and systematic consideration, there is a similar need for informed debate about nearly three-quarters of elderly people in the UK who live separately from younger people. Of course, these figures unhelpfully group together millions of fit elderly people whose life-style differs little from when they were middle aged. Nonetheless, a high proportion of those who live beyond 75 will suffer a degree of frailty, ill-health or disability which makes them dependent on external sources of support for their comfort and well-being. Whether it is available and adequate will no doubt have some bearing on the growth of residential care.

The balance in this country between old people in private households and those in residential care is not sacred or immutable. Other countries, such as The Netherlands, have different traditions which have resulted in a much higher proportion of old people in residential care. Later (Chapter 6), we consider some of the strengths and weaknesses, potential and actual, of residential care. However, most would accept that ideally elderly people should have a choice of agreeable alternatives to suit their circumstances and conditions and that a majority would choose to remain in their own homes. A flight to residential care from a disagreeable home situation cannot be described as choice.

What then does care *by* the community imply for those who choose to live *in* it? The relationship between informal and formal systems is a critical issue. In the care of the very old people living in independent households, informal systems will rarely be wholly sufficient. This is at variance with some of the sentimentalised exaggerations, conveniently associated with cost saving, about the role and scope of informal care.

Therefore, a starting point for any discussion of community care must be a realistic appraisal of informal systems.

Informal carers are comprised of relatives, friends and neighbours. There is no dispute that relatives, or 'kin', are the primary source of support for old people at home. Relatives carry out various caring activities, from physical care to a wide range of less intimate but crucial household tasks. They offer to their old people many opportunities for social interaction and for emotionally rewarding experiences. Any suggestion that this level of care is diminishing is not borne out in the findings of numerous studies. Indeed, an old person living alone may need nearly as much physical care as those in shared households and this may require quite a high level of family organisation and planning, in which a woman is usually at the centre. Such support, however, has to be seen in the context of changing family patterns and of the patterns of employment. Discussion of family support often seems to assume geographical propinquity, which is increasingly problematic. The present and future impact of unemployment on the well-being of old people has yet to be assessed and indeed may be most strongly felt in the next decade or two. In fact, we have little solid evidence of the effects of earlier waves of unemployment on old people. Yet common observation suggests that some of today's isolated old people suffer in part from the consequences of those periods of dislocation. A predictable consequence of long-term rising unemployment, unless there is a widespread economic decline, is that first men, and then families, move in search of work, usually leaving elderly people behind. At the point of departure, when young middle aged children are most likely to seek work, their parents are often fit and future problems do not loom large. The elderly people may have a range of social connections which would understandably be given up with reluctance and they often do not at that stage need to give up their home. Yet, since family remains the prime source of close personal care, ten years on the situation may become precarious and fraught with practical and social complications. Apart from immediate logistical difficulties, the natural links of reciprocity may be weakened over the years by geographical distance so that a natural and gradual change in the balance between dependence and independence has not been effected. If, therefore, an old person at this stage moves a distance into the son or daughter's home, they may not only lose a lifetime of familiar associations but they must struggle with complex adjustments within the family.

This analysis is not unfamiliar; such situations are common amongst middle class families whose occupational and geographical mobility has been greater than that of the working class. However, the rise of unemployment creates a particular problem for the next generation of 'very old', whose numbers are in any case increasing. Furthermore, working class old people left behind in areas of deprivation, where the economic recession has bitten hard, may face difficulties of a quite different kind from their middle class counterparts. Urban decay brings with it a host of associated miseries which impact especially severely on old people. We are now all familiar with the sadness and anxieties of old people left in derelict streets, taken over by those whom they fear. In short, we have not as yet experienced the full extent of the social dislocation consequent upon this period of unemployment. For those who work in certain parts of the country, it will be severe and prolonged. It is a matter to which statutory services in those areas most affected should be paying serious attention now, since adverse effects on old people's support systems are predictable.

The ripples of family disturbance which unemployment brings are spread widely too amongst those who do not move away from their home area. The consequences for the old are sad: on a practical level, when income is restricted, all kinds of practical and material benefits may also be denied to old people. Sympathy is often centred upon the younger family, little is said about its indirect effects on old people, who themselves are often reluctant to complain. Yet one has only to think (for example) about giving up a car, to see how significant the effects on an old person may be, in terms of contact with their relatives and services offered. It is one of the many ironies in our provision for old people that we offer the fit elderly cheap transport (which they take up enthusiastically to visit their relatives) but make no provision to enable the relatives of the frail housebound to visit them. The cost of bus fares for a family to visit their grandmother takes a disproportionate slice out of an income support (formerly supplementary benefit) Giro.

Social dislocation, of course, is not simply a function of unemployment. There has been considerable comment, usually negative, about the waves of elderly people who in retirement moved away from their home town to a supposedly more agreeable environment, the south coast for example. It is not clear whether that fashion persists or whether tales of 'geriatric ghettos' and overstretched services have reached the next generation. It also remains to be seen whether better preretirement and health education programmes will play a part in helping people prepare constructively for old age and to make a realistic appraisal of the matters which are and will be of greater importance to them than sea air.

Thus, the effects of unemployment and associated poverty in the younger generation bear hardly (and will increasingly do so) upon one especially vulnerable section of the elderly population, further depriving a group whose own material and financial disadvantage is striking. Others may find contact with kin more difficult because they have moved. As discussed in the previous chapter, relationships with kin will also be affected by the higher incidence of divorce and remarriage, which may weaken the support available to the old living alone, especially because, in such interactions, the notion of reciprocity over time is so important.

The fact that an increasing number of women want paid employment has also placed further strain on caring arrangements. Frequently, this is part-time and is managed – albeit with difficulty – alongside other family respon-sibilities. Hours of work may be difficult to reconcile with the needs of the old person. The attitude of employers to domestic responsibilities is of consider-able importance and highly variable. In general, there is less understanding extended to those with 'parent care' problems than 'child care' problems, despite the power of the social assumption that it is 'women's work'.

As with care within the household, the provision of care from outside can be a formidable task. Although less stressful in one sense than the 24-hour care of a relative at home, in another way it can be more stressful. These domestic arrangements may depend on a number of people 'pulling their weight' and the reliability of individuals is critical for the safety and well-being of the old person. (A teenager who forgets to call in at the appointed time may cause real distress.) Futhermore, the fact that the old person is alone, especially at night, is a con-stant source of anxiety. In all this, women, usually middle aged, continue to play the major part. They are often keenly aware of the familial conflict that this produces. How to please everybody remains a central motif in many women's lives and the source of quite powerful feelings of oppression.

This kind of family care is not merely between parents and succeeding generations of children. Indeed, a significant number of very old people have no younger surviving children, as Mark Abrams (1978, 1980) showed in his Age Concern surveys.

This has major implications for those who develop and provide services. For such old people, other relatives are sometimes available. For example, a substantial number of siblings, even cousins, are involved in these inter-actions as Wenger (1984) has shown. But for many old people, being without children is a significant factor in loneliness and isolation.

Wenger's study of a rural community in Wales reminds us that, in some relatively stable areas, systems of such informal care seem adequate to meet a very high proportion of elderly people's needs. Whether that holds true for very frail old people is doubtful as Wenger herself recognises. We should nonetheless acknowledge that in some parts of the country family care is extensive and durable.

Friends are another source of informal support. This has been subjected to critical scrutiny by Allan (1986). In a sharp analysis, Allan claims that

> there is very little empirical evidence that friends actually do provide very much long term care of the form envisaged in community care policies.

Allan argues that the very nature of friendship is one of equality and recipro-city and that this will impose limits on what it is acceptable to give or to receive.

> The equality on which the relationship is premised breaks down. Friend-ships ... are not particularly durable. Over time, they alter and change. ... In particular, most friendships do not endure when the circumstances of one of the friends is altered in any major fashion.

With regard to elderly people, Allan suggests that, in any case, old people have for a variety of reasons quite small friendship circles and that even within those circles

> it is still far from obvious that these will prove particularly suitable for any significant level of care provision ... receiving assistance from the other without any acceptable means of reciprocation is quite contrary to the way most friendships are routinely ordered.

Finally, Allan draws a distinction between different forms of caring and sug-gests that 'tending' is usually outside the range of tasks which friends would perform. Friendship is more likely to be offered in terms of emotional support or help in times of crisis.

There is much in Allan's discussion which accords with everyday experi-ence. Yet friendship patterns and their significance vary greatly between different groups in society, in particular between men and women, different social classes, and the single, the married and widowed. One should therefore be cautious about generalisations which do less than justice to the contribu-tion which friendship can make to the well-being of specific groups of old

people. This is well illustrated by Jerrome (1981) who ex⸱....ned the significance of friendship for middle class women in later life. She concluded that

> for the women in the study, friendship both given and received gives
> meaning to existence and a structure to life in retirement.

However, Jerrome's findings do not refer at all to 'tending' activities; the
importance of friends in old age seems to be more about a natural extension of
satisfying experiences and modes of behaviour in earlier years than about a
changed conception of the nature of the relationship which could accommodate more 'caring' activity. Although there will be significant exceptions, and
these should be further studied, friendship is not a primary vehicle for the
provision of the care that so many old people need.

Finally, in this consideration of informal care outside the home, we turn to
neighbours.

Philip Abrams, who died tragically young in 1981, spent a number of
extremely productive years researching the nature of neighbourliness and the
relationship of informal to formal care systems. Extensive use is made here in
this chapter of his posthumously published work (Bulmer, 1986) because it
has so much to say of immediate and striking significance to our theme.

In Abrams' definition, neighbours are simply people who

> live near one another; neighbouring 'is the actual pattern of interaction'
> which can be perceived negatively or positively, whereas 'neighbour-
> liness' is 'a positive and committed relationship constructed between
> neighbours'. Neighbourhoods, it should be noted, will probably be
> defined differently by local people and service providers!   (Bulmer, 1986)

Abrams attempted to account for some of the striking variations in 'neighbour
behaviour' which he found in different areas. Even to list these begins to
unravel some of the complications in this everyday concept. He described first
'foreground factors'; these include how long people have lived in an area and
how settled it is; how close people are physically; and the age and stage in the
lifecycle and gender: Abrams comments that:

> segregation of the elderly in bungalows ... and flats ... cuts them off
> from neighbours other than people of their own age and accentuated
> their isolation.

To mothers with young children and the elderly, neighbours assumed special
importance; women, especially in working class areas, were more neighbourly than men. Background factors further elaborate the variations. Personal history was very important, in creating expectations of how neighbours
should behave. Social class was highly significant:

> Middle class residents had a different role and a different relationship to
> their neighbour. Their range of social contacts was wider, friends and
> relatives more likely to be geographically distant.

Yet this behaviour was related to wider trends than simply social class; it concerned the balance between closeness and distance, and the nature of support networks. Leaving kin aside (and many are neighbours), Abrams pointed out that many modern neighbours have no basis for interdependence other than proximity. They are not linked in other ways, as they might have been in the past, as in mining villages, by other common bonds of interests. Such conclusions, drawn from detailed analyses of the views and attitudes of people in different parts of the country, present those who plan services with an immediate challenge – the need to understand the dynamics of 'neighbouring' in their own localities. These can vary dramatically within quite small geographical areas. Such understanding is necessary, not simply to assess realistically what can and cannot be expected of such informal care, but also to develop the formal sector of care in a way which takes account of the prevailing norms of a given area.

At the heart of much of the debate about neighbourliness lie questions about reciprocity and altruism. Much neighbourly activity is clearly reciprocal – mutual and balanced exchange is at the core of the relationships day by day. This is clearly not the case where some very frail old people are concerned but reciprocity can be viewed over a long time scale. Thus, as do relatives, neighbours may reciprocate for care offered many years ago ('she was very good to us as children; she was very good to mother').

Obviously, the existence of such ties and their translation into present day activity is dependent on geographical and social stability. It is perhaps surprising that it has survived at all, yet there are pockets in this country where these lifetime associations are still meaningful.

In any case, the importance of reciprocating has to be set beside other motivations which may underpin neighbourly acts as well as those in various forms of voluntary service. The concept of altruism has been much discussed. Abrams (Bulmer, 1986) drew attention to the complexity of the concept; many who are perceived as altruistic will themselves acknowledge the profound satisfaction which they derive from their supposedly selfless activities but find it difficult to put this into words. We need not here dwell long on these matters. Fortunately for frail elderly people, there are many who offer altruistic neighbouring acts, that is to say, they are done without assumptions of reciprocity; the gratification which they obtain is in a sense their own private business! However, because so much 'neighbouring' has been rooted in the notion of mutual exchange, and has always involved a fine balance between closeness and distance, it is in some ways harder for the parties to adapt to a changed role than it is, for example, in a situation where the supporter is defined from the outset as a voluntary visitor.

In any case, there are usually distinctions drawn by neighbour and old person alike concerning the nature of the activity which it is appropriate to offer and to accept. Thus, shopping is a regular feature of neighbourly support but intimate bodily tasks are rarely performed. Money matters are a delicate area; pensions may be cashed but discussion of an old person's financial problems may be considered inappropriate. Such boundaries have to be respected for they mirror deeply entrenched attitudes and social expectations. Nor are the expectations of neighbouring necessarily mutually understood by those living beside each other. In areas of geographical mobility people may be neighbours who are culturally strangers. Inner cities with mixed ethnic groupings are an example. Younger neighbours are often very concerned about these old neighbours. On the one hand, there is lifelong caution about intrusiveness. Abrams remarked

> we have been impressed by the degree to which the desire to help is inhibited in practice by a reluctance to intrude oneself into other people's lives.

On the other hand, the vulnerability of such old people creates considerable anxiety. There is also fear of involvement which could become burdensome, especially since many neighbours will have their own worries about relatives. On occasion, old people are difficult to help and neighbourly relations become fraught. A particular, and not infrequent, problem arises when mental infirmity leads old people to behave in ways which are difficult for neighbours to tolerate.

What of the future? Abrams argued that traditional neighbourliness will not survive and that its passing is not to be deplored, because it was so often a reaction to adverse social conditions.

> Reciprocal care between neighbours grows where information and trust are high and where resources for satisfying needs in other ways are low, in relatively isolated, relatively closed and relatively threatened social milieu with highly homogeneous populations. . . . Traditional informal networks are dying and should be allowed to die.

These networks, which included certain kinds of neigbouring, included those for whom ties of kinship were of primary significance. There is ample evidence that those ties remain strong even as the character of networks changes in other ways and thus these basic family links continue to be the first line of defence, the more so because other forms of association may weaken. However, that the strain on some families, especially female members, is thus increased is indisputable and makes the case for complementary support, through organised local endeavour, all the more compelling.

Abrams argued that in place of traditional informal networks, one can observe the growth of '*neighbourhoodism*', which is 'an attempt by new-comers to create a local social world through political or quasi political action'. He referred to 'the success of the enormous diversity of neighbourhood Care Projects up and down the country (which) springs from these sources'.

Neighbourhood care today means working out a constructive relationship between the state, locally and nationally, and neighbourhoodism, the politicised voice of local attachment.

If we cling to an outmoded view of neighbouring, peering at it through deeply rose-tinted spectacles, we may make false assumptions about what is actually available to old people, or ought to be available. We may seek to recreate care arrangements which no longer have within them the seeds of growth. Where they still exist, it is important that they are not undermined; but where they have withered away, we need to look to new models which take account of the changing patterns and forces in modern society. This is, however, problematic for old people. Abrams referred to greater mobility and greater choice as weakening the traditional neighbour's ties. Unfortunately, this further emphasises the separateness of old people (not dissimilar to mothers of young children) precisely because they so often do not share in this extended range of opportunities and are more dependent on what is locally available. One should not therefore underestimate the importance of *neighbourhood* to such old people, even if *neighbours* do not perform the same functions as in 'the old days'. One relevant finding of Abrams' research was that in successful neighbourhood care there were often central figures, key individuals, perceived as critical to the scheme.

> They are . . . the people whose position and activities enable them to fuse and mediate both neighbourhood involvement and social services care. . . .

They often already occupied formal roles in the area – doctors, priests, post-mistresses or teachers, which reminds us of the ways in which informal and formal roles and structures interact. This perceived competence in one role leading to the acquisition of other roles, brings us, in concluding this discussion of informal care, to one of Abrams' most telling points, for those who want to place such neighbourly care in a contemporary context. It was noted that to engage in such activities, people needed to feel that they had special areas of competence whether, for example, in knowing how to lift people, in tending the dying, and in knowing your way round the system. People who did not know how to be useful dropped out of Good Neighbour schemes. The implications for those who wish to mobilise modern-style informal care are obvious.

In what has been described, we have moved from a model of a community in which neighbourly acts were performed within clearly defined limits, with reciprocal benefits looming large, to a model in which, so far as very old people are concerned, such acts are more often the product of altruism (remembering that this does not deny gratification to the giver) and of a more systematic attempt to offer and channel care appropriately. Of course, that leaves us with the problem raised in the first chapter – the extent to which such old people feel they are no longer able to engage in transactions which benefit others as well as themselves. How far that can be mitigated by more sensitive evaluation of the distinctive contribution individual old people may have still to make, should be one of the questions for all workers in this field to address as they go about their daily work.

CHAPTER 4

Care in the community II: Caring and tending

The word 'carer' has come into common usage in the past ten years or so, but it has been used imprecisely. There are two aspects of its definition to which we must first give attention. Firstly, *who* does it describe; secondly, *what* does it describe?

As Oliver (1986) has recently pointed out, the word was originally used in respect of those who cared for dependent adult relatives, mostly elderly people:

> It meant a person who was not paid, was probably a close relative and had a strong emotional involvement with the person receiving care.

But this has been widened, to Oliver's regret. She notes that 'social workers, foster parents, foster families for olderly people, care assistants . . . nursing auxilliaries, privately employed housekeepers' are now described as carers. Oliver regards the distinction between paid and unpaid as critical and argues 'let us have our word back'!

From the perspective of those who seek to draw political and social attention to a group who have been much exploited and little supported, the objection to widening the use of the term is understandable. And there certainly are major differences between the groups of people to whom the term is now applied. However, there are some important similarities to which attention also needs to be drawn, especially in relation to the second aspect of the definition, *what* it describes.

Parker's (1981) contribution to the debate, in his introduction of the word 'tending', is now widely used and is helpful. The term 'caring' is too wide to have much utility and the use of 'tending' as an element of caring has made it clear that the focus is upon those who perform physical tasks for others. The horticultural overtone is not unattractive; we 'tend' the plants in the garden and the term to a gardener implies more than supplying their basic needs. Gardeners respect and understand the characteristics of their plants. One even hears that plants respond to the spoken word! 'Tend' is a gentle word.

Such tending, of course, is provided by both the paid and the unpaid. We consider some of the implications for paid carers in Chapter 7. Oliver is right, however, to insist that the crucial issue of the unpaid carer should not be lost in more general comment and it is upon this we concentrate here.

Unpaid carers, in the context of the present discussion, are in three main categories. There are old people, spouses and other relatives, caring for each other; middle aged or 'younger' elderly people, mostly women, caring for the old; and a variety of relatives, neighbours and friends, not in the same household, who perform some tending activities.

In a recent paper, Arber *et al.* (1986) presented some data based upon an analysis of the *General Household Survey*. They analyse the household structure in which elderly people live, by gender of the elderly person and percentage of the severely disabled. Arber *et al.* argue that some important issues have been clouded by a failure in the literature to distinguish between the two different types of household structure: old living with old, and younger living with old. It is argued that those, especially feminists, who stress the exploitation of women as carers have failed to take account of the significant numbers of men in the first category.

> Male carers are often omitted from detailed study because they are seen to be unimportant or assumed to be so few in number. A fuller understanding of the differences and similarities between male and female carers is long overdue . . .

Arber *et al.* used the *General Household Survey* of 1980, which provides a nationally representative sample of over 4500 elderly persons in private households to study patterns of care in households in which there were severely disabled people.

> Apart from the elderly living alone, married couples predominate as the type of household containing elderly people in need of care. . . . Over half the severely disabled elderly are living only with the spouse and exactly half the spouses caring for an elderly disabled partner are men.

Twelve per cent of the elderly disabled live with one or more 'single' elderly. The majority of these are elderly women, many of whom are caring for siblings. As Arber *et al.* note, in both these groups,

> the nature of the caring relationship is likely to be based on love and mutual support over a long period of time. The elderly partners may have varying degrees of disability and, at any one time, the more able may be the primary carer, but this may shift over time and with variation in the physical health of each partner. These may be characterised as fragile caring units of mutual support.

Although those who work with old people will have observed for themselves that in this group there are a significant number of male carers, the implications have not been fully drawn out because so many old disabled people at home alone are women and so many younger women carry the main burden of informal care at home. (The former is, of course, a reflection of the greater longevity of women, often left alone after bereavement.) Arber *et al.* use this data to challenge some of the widely cited research findings from the Equal Opportunities Commission (1984), that men carers receive a disproportionate share of the statutory services. It must be stressed that the data is complex and bound up with difficulties of defining levels of disability, different kind of household and service, and dependent upon sophisticated statistical analysis. However, their conclusion will come as a surprise to many who eagerly espoused the work of the EOC. They state that:

> ... evidence of discrimination was primarily on the basis of type of household and the marital status of the carer rather than on the gender of the carer. ... (Domiciliary) services appear to be provided where no family is available rather than to assist a family in their support.
>
> (Arber *et al.*, 1986)

We shall consider the position of younger carers later. So far as the old, mutually dependent carers are concerned, this work is valuable in reminding us of the substantial numbers of men who perform these functions for their wives. It shows, unequivocally, that many men in the last years of their lives do assume roles and perform tasks which have been traditionally associated with women, and it is clear that a substantial number do so with skill and tenderness. It reminds us of the adaptability of old people about which earlier comment has been made and suggests that the rigid divisions between the sexes in tending roles, although still powerful, may not be so impermeable as they sometimes appear. Such reflections do not, of course, address an even more fundamental question – should old spouses, or those otherwise related, of either sex, have to do so much for each other?

We must be cautious how we answer. As Levin *et al.* (1983) have so clearly shown, many of those who perform such roles want support, and a measure of relief, but they do not wish to abdicate what they perceive as their responsibility. There is a danger, however, that such generalisations are used to disguise significant variations in the reaction to the position in which old people have been placed. For example, long-standing marital disharmony may lie behind apparent rejection; indeed, it may be that the disability of one partner provides the first and only reliable opportunity for old people to separate. Also, for all carers, older or younger, the ability to tolerate *specific* aspects of their partner's behaviour is a significant factor. For example, faecal incontinence and sleep disturbance are often associated with the breakdown of caring arrangements leading to hospitalisation. Long-standing patterns of marital and familial interaction also play a part in the nature of the dependence that is developed, and the extent to which, within the constraints of the situation, it is mutually satisfying. How easy or how difficult does a partner find it to give or to receive physical care? These are matters to which we alluded in Chapter 2. For married couples, it seems likely that it will be to an extent related to the degree of easy intimacy which they have achieved in sexual relations. Nor should the continuing need for sexual relationships be overlooked. There is a strong tendency to belittle or ignore sexual activity in old age, but the feelings of carers may be affected by the degree of frustration experienced in that aspect of life.

In this connection, it should be remembered that a proportion of elderly partnerships will be gay or lesbian. It is one of the enduring sadnesses of people in such relationships that they are not offered the same respect and sympathy as man and wife. Other relatives and professionals collude in ignoring what they in fact know – that these people have lived together sexually, domestically and financially as if they were married. Their distress and sadness about the predicament of their partner will be no different although it may be concealed from others by awkwardness about their sexual preference. In old age, however, the likelihood is that the overwhelming need will be for confirmation and acceptance of their situation.

We have spoken about old partners as if they will always have had a long life together and that is indeed the case in many of the pairs whom we currently encounter. However, post-war, the rise in divorce rates and remarriage, peaking in the 1970s, means that we shall in future meet more old people whose relationships may not have been lifelong. One can only speculate on the implications of that for the last years of life and, in particular, for the acceptance of tending roles.

Amongst the 'old carers', as has already been indicated, there are a substantial number of siblings, especially sisters. In such cases, special factors are at work, particularly as physical dependence increases, which relate to the experiences of childhood. Such old people may have little embarrassment with each other about bodily functions, perhaps less than some husbands and wives because they were the stuff of taken-for-granted childhood. They may also show in their relationships past patterns of control and authority, together with assumptions about each other, sometimes resented, based on years of family labelling ('Meg is the extravagant one'). Nor should it be assumed that siblings who have lived apart, sometimes married, for many years have broken these profound childhood links which shaped their attitudes to each other.

When one begins to explore such aspects of old people's mutual care, the need for help which goes beyond the provision of practical support is obvious. There are worlds of feeling to be gently explored in seeking to provide what is really needed. On occasion, the need to separate and the guilt about it may be the focus of work; more often, it will be to validate and confirm the spouse or partner in the activities which they are performing. For this kind of caring is often seen as the dignified proper response to long years of partnership and is realistically faced as a price that can be gladly paid for past happiness. Along with that acceptance must also go the acknowledgement of intimations of morality – 'who will go first?'. It is not uncommon for the carer to fear that they may predecease their partner, who will thus be deserted. These are matters which, with due regard to the personal privacy of those who have been together so long, may need to be aired, sometimes in the context of plans for the future.

The second major groups of carers to which we now turn are the younger (usually) relatives caring for an elderly disabled member of the household. About 70 per cent of those elderly persons living with younger people are severely disabled. The proportion amongst the very old will be even higher. Quite different household patterns are involved. In particular, there is a distinction between those adult children, often single, of old people, who have lived with them long before the dependency arose and those, often married, who offer a home to an old parent hitherto living independently. It is obvious that these are very different situations in which different issues and problems arise. With regard to the former,

> as the elderly person becomes older, the situation is likely to change from one in which the able-bodied parent primarily provides servicing to the younger single adult . . . to one in which the relationship is primarily one of dependency.   (Arber *et al.*, 1986)

We know little of how this relationship changes over time. From the Arber analysis, it appears that 'single women are performing a caring role to a greater extent than men'. But it should be noted that a substantial minority (45 per cent) of single adults caring for such parents were male.

We have little evidence from research as to how the members of such households view the changing balance of the relationship. The dependency of the old person may emerge gradually with increasing frailty or suddenly, as after a stroke. The adult parent, usually the mother, may have provided the main domestic support for a working son or daughter over many years. Indeed, as Evers (1984) found in her study, old people who in objective terms may be described as severely disabled may continue to perform these services, such as preparing the evening meal, and many function domestically more competently than those who are less physically impaired. This is, of course, bound up with the personalities and attitudes of the persons concerned and the history of their relationships. As Arber *et al.* (1986) remark, however, there may be 'serious conflicting demands between the demands of caring and the carer's paid employment and social activities'. They may need a good deal of support because of these conflicts, yet this is rarely available. For many, the critical point in the conflict will revolve around giving up work. Paradoxically, the availability of the Invalid Care Allowance (until recently restricted to single carers) may sharpen the dilemma, for if some alternative financial support is available (albeit not generous) giving up work becomes a real possibility. Yet for many employment offers social satisfaction as great or greater than the financial reward.

Those who argue for a 'carer's benefit' need to ponder this point and consider ways in which such allowances could be used to support the existing arrangements in a household in which carers are in employment and wish to continue. (This would, of course, imply an allowance which was not means-tested as is the Invalid Care Allowance.) However, a substantial number of the carers in this category are in fact over retirement age. Indeed, it is not unusual for someone recently retired (and perhaps looking forward to it) to find themselves coping with sharply increasing dependency of their parents and unable to enjoy the period of active leisure which they were anticipating.

Whilst it has been made clear that in this group both men and women assume caring roles, feminists have rightly pointed out that some of the dilemmas and problems are worse for women, not least because social conventions have not ascribed the same significance to employment for women as for men. Finch and Groves (1983) provide a compelling account of some of the difficulties which women encounter. Their focus is 'upon the tension between women's . . . independence (actual, potential or desired) and their traditional role as front line unpaid carers'. Wright (Finch and Groves, 1983) reports a small survey of single carers from which women were more likely to have given up employment than men in order to care for parents, sometimes giving up secure and well paid work when in their late forties or earlier fifties. The implications of this for their future as well as their present financial circumstances are obvious. Others in the survey had reduced their hours of work or made special arrangements. Many years ago, I had the opportunity to read and report on the position of a group of such women who were on Supplementary Benefit. The picture painted of the isolation and constriction of their lives was profoundly depressing. Poverty was not experienced as a problem because there was so little that women wanted to spend money on ('No, I don't go out in the evenings, Mother doesn't like it.' 'No I don't get my hair done, it's not worth it'). It is reassuring to note that the burden which such women carry has been more widely recognised and discussed in the past 10–15 years. For this, those feminists, such as Finch and Groves (1983), who espoused the cause of their older sisters, can take some credit, particularly in the challenge they threw down to those who assumed without question that such roles would naturally fall to women on their own.

The numbers of single (i.e. unmarried) women, have fallen significantly in recent years, with important consequences for the caring professions as well as informal care. However, it remains to be seen whether in their place will arise a significant number of women who have married, divorced and not remarried and to whom society would wish to ascribe similar roles. If so, it is to be hoped that their contribution to support of old people, and their need for support themselves, will be more sensitively and generously appraised than in the past. Two aspects of caring in these circumstances stand out; firstly, the loneliness, especially when, as is common, the old person is demented. The experience of daily living with someone whose 'mind is gone' is peculiarly bleak, almost unimaginable (yet we must try) for those who have not experienced it. Secondly, the burden of *detail* in daily care can be nearly overwhelming. Where extreme physical dependence is present, every aspect of daily living has to be planned and managed. Every journey from bed to bathroom, from sitting room to kitchen is a hazard. Every event, dressing, mealtimes and so on, must be a sequence of carefully organised activities to make the process easier, indeed, manageable at all. Of course, this applies to all carers of the very frail. But because this group of people is isolated, the routines may assume a particularly tedious, inexorable character. Small wonder if tempers are sometimes frayed and words or actions rough. These are the women who cry alone at night. And life for their male counterparts may be no less bleak.

Turning now to consider the other main group of younger household carers, there are an increasing number, currently about 11 per cent, of elderly people living with younger people, usually daughters and sons-in-law. There is wide agreement that, in such households, it is women who take the main share of responsibility. The work of Nissel and Bonnerjea (1982) has been widely cited and, although a small survey, its findings have not been seriously contested. They have indeed been confirmed by others such as Abrams and Marsden (1986), and most recently, by Lewis and Meredith (1988) (to whom we refer later). A distinctive and particularly valuable aspect of the study by Nissel and Bonnerjea was the keeping of diaries by their respondents so that they could describe the nature of, and measure the time taken in, the caring activities undertaken. Although not in a sense surprising, the impact of the bare facts is nonetheless considerable: for it emerged that these women spent an average of over three hours on weekdays on various caring activities compared to the 13 minutes offered by men! (These averages, of course, conceal substantial discrepancies according to the need of the relative.) Perhaps even more significant, well over half of the husbands played *no* direct part in caring. Moreover, the picture that emerges is of very considerable feelings of isolation, even within a marital couple. There was a surprising lack of help from other relatives, which Nissel and Bonnerjea suggest should be further explored elsewhere. They point to the difficulties which some carers experience in getting help from informal sources with particular forms of disability, especially for people with severe mental infirmity and incontinence. They single out 'tension in the family' as 'a theme which runs through the interviews in a variety of forms'.

> There is often disagreement between spouses; wives complain at best about lack of help and support from their husbands, at worst that their husbands make increased demands and take out their frustrations about the relative on their wives; husbands complain that their wives are so

tired that they cannot have a decent conversation, dinner or social night out.

The study identified the main sources of difficulty in the family reactions. One was the complaint of lack of privacy. A second was the emergence of a triangular relationship with the woman as 'pig in the middle'; a particular point of concern was that the 'majority of husbands gave the impression of being quite distant from the situation'. Children were less directly affected but there were considerable indirect effects, in terms of the time their mothers had for them and the effect of the grandparent on daily living. (The actual numbers of such three-generational households are very small, about two per cent. However, implications for particular families may nonetheless be considerable.)

Amongst the carers themselves, 'isolation, frustration and resignation' were near universal in the sample, with a substantial number estimating that their sense of self-worth had suffered as a result of their situation. This was partly due to loss of employment or employment prospects but, as indicated above, they may begin to accept 'being a nobody and start acting in a way that confirms the label. . . . They stop buying new clothes or wearing make up' and so on. Nissell and Bonnerjea acutely observe that all this may lead to 'a lack of perspective on the situation' so that they may find it difficult to accept appropriate help or place limits on their involvement.

Despite the small numbers involved, this work has been discussed at some length because the issues raised are critical for all those who work with elderly people and carers. Many of their findings and conclusions are supported in the recent study by Lewis and Meredith (1988), in which the sample comprised both single and married women. The work of Abrams and Marsden (1986) strikingly, and it must be said depressingly, confirms the impression given by earlier studies. Abrams and Marsden interviewed 38 such women caring for mothers aged 75 or over who were living with them. The bleak conclusion of the study is that:

> In general . . . rejection *appears* to increase with the development of disability and the continuation of caring . . . only a handful of these disabled mothers would be said to be receiving tending in a context which was predominantly loving . . .

> The association between the daughters rejection and the mother's disability *appears* to afford at least circumstantial evidence that relationships deteriorate as a consequence of the burdens of tending.

Abrams and Marsden open up an important and neglected aspect of this question – the impact of social class upon attitudes to caring. They suggest that:

> there was something about these middle class daughter's relationships with their (rather *less*) disabled mothers which made sharing a household less tolerable to them than for working class daughters.

These matters remain further to be explored. Another important finding of the study was the confusion and ambivalence which these carers exhibited in relation to role reversal. Were they now mothering their own mothers, and if they were, did they resent it? The authors suggest that

> in over half of the households with severely incapacitated mothers, it was the breakdown in personal interaction and reciprocity which the daughters found most distressing, burdensome and hard to take.

They add that the impact of the mother's presence on the marriage may have caused further resentment. It is not impossible that the situation is harder to tolerate in these households than in those with single carers. The implications of such evidence for family social policy are extensive and disturbing. The state depends on these relationships for the support of the vast majority of severely disabled old people. If a sizeable proportion of these are characterised by extreme ambivalence, even hostility, it throws into question many assumptions about this form of community care as preferable to (say) residential care.

Lewis and Meredith (1988) reveal similar tensions and problems although the picture which they draw is less bleak, showing a number of women whose recollections of caring for their mothers are predominantly positive, even if stressful. This study breaks new ground in drawing on the women's memories of the caring experience once it is over. The impressions gained are therefore not 'snapshots' but the distillation of an experience often spread over many years and with distinct phases. Furthermore, this is one of the few studies which gives an account of the feelings after the task was completed. It suggests the unmet need of so many women for support and help in redefining their role and purpose when the all-consuming daily tending of another is no longer required.

In Chapter 8, issues arising from the presence in this country of substantial ethnic minorities will be discussed. In the present context of 'tending', two points should be noted. Firstly, because there are wide variations between different ethnic groups in the time of arrival in this country and their age on entry, the numbers of those who have reached advanced years, in general small, differs greatly between groups. Thus, for example, there are substantial numbers of very old Jews, comparatively few very old Asians. The need for 'tending' varies accordingly. Secondly, there are also wide variations between groups in the extent to which care *within* families is available. Those who came as refugees from Europe have sometimes lost their families, through death or migration to other parts of the world. They may be quite isolated. Others, such as Asians, may be at present living within extended families. For example, one research study cited by Mays (1983) suggested that only about 5 per cent of Asian elders live alone (compared with 38 per cent of white old people) (Bhalla and Blakemore, 1981). Furthermore, 56 per cent lived in households with between five and eight people, whereas, nationally, only about 2 per cent of white old people live in three-generation households.

These illustrations are simply suggestive of the complexities which are likely to be involved when we attempt to understand patterns of 'tending' within families of different cultural background. Furthermore, as Mays (1983) remarks, the 'limited evidence of changing attitudes of family patterns . . . needs to be tested more thoroughly'. It is all too easy to fall into the stereotypical trap, on the one hand, of assuming the continuance of traditional patterns and, on the other, of predicting their total breakdown! For practitioners, the most important issue is to seek to understand the norms of behaviour within different groups and the extent to which these are challenged, modified or overturned by families living in contemporary Britain, whose social and economic circumstances are vastly different from those which pertained in their land of origin. In particular the significance of gender in relation to tending activities merits sensitive exploration.

What, then, do we make of the substantial and growing literature on informal carers? There would seem to be three points of especial significance.

1. Carers are not a homogeneous group. Tending takes place in a wide variety of households, characterised by different family structures and by widely different experiences in terms of family relationships and life patterns. This has particular importance in relation to ethnic minorities. Research so far has only begun to offer sociological or psychological analyses which would enable us to develop typologies of carers and those cared for.

2. There is a need to recognise and further consider the position of male carers, while not using this issue to deflect us from the more general issues which arise for women through entrenched assumptions that this is their 'natural' role.

3. The factors which lead to breakdown in such caring, and in particular to the emergence of a predominantly rejecting relationship, are still imperfectly understood. We need to be clearer about the interactions which affect this, and whether there are substantially more breakdowns when mental infirmity, especially dementia, is present in old people, or whether other factors are of equal significance.

Behind much of the discussions about tending lie complex questions concerning social attitudes and values ascribed to the provision of physical care for other human beings. (This, of course, applies to paid as well as unpaid carers.)

There is a profound hypocrisy in society on these matters. Although value is ascribed to the caring expressive functions, especially those of motherhood, it is frequently of a somewhat sentimental and patronising kind. That is to say, hymns of praise are sung, especially to mothers, but the tangible rewards which might be expected for work of considerable social significance are not available. Since this is inextricably bound up with women's position in society as the prime providers of such tending, it becomes difficult to say whether the depressed status of such work is a result of a system of male domination of women or whether such work has been allocated to women as part of that process. However that may be, this hypocrisy has one profoundly disturbing consequence. It invites denigration, even denial, of the link between physical care and care for the whole person whose body needs tending, and therefore of the knowledge and skill which such activities may require.

In contemporary British society this link is accepted to a greater degree so far as the care of children and motherhood is concerned, though social attitudes still reveal some of the same ambivalence. Here the influences of the professionals, psychologists, psychiatrists, psycho-analysts and paediatricians have played an important part in convincing us (as every mother knows) that the quality of physical care has a profound effect on the social and emotional development of children. Of course, this can be, and has been, used to 'lock' women in the home environment. Yet at least there are profound gratifications for many women from the assumption of the role which is acknowledged as socially valuable, in the contribution it makes to the health and well-being of the next generation. It offers immediate and intense psychological satisfaction to many women.

The position of those who tend the very old is much less assured, in terms of the social values ascribed to the activity. Again social messages are confused: home helps, for example, are frequently praised, yet their wages, like those of care assistants, do not offer practical confirmation of that praise. (It is interesting to see that recent union negotiations may place the wages of such workers above those of refuse collectors for the first time.) Similar problems arise, of course, in the care of other groups who need tending, such as the profoundly handicapped. But the sheer numbers of very old people who depend on informal and formal 'tenders' make this issue of great social significance – and increasingly so. Furthermore, unlike the care of children, the personal rewards are not as obvious and, in some cases, may be non-existent or hard to define.

In contrast to care of children, those who tend the very old have no unequivocal proof of their success in terms of a healthy developing body. Confirmation of the value of the activity lies in prevention and alleviation of discomfort and in the responses of those for whom they care. Their rewards are ultimately humanitarian. Of course, those who provide such care in the context of a lifetime of love have another frame of reference upon which to draw for satisfaction. This may be vital in making tolerable those activities which are stressful and distasteful. In these situations it is often the deterioration of the mind of the old person which makes tending tasks so hard to bear, which reminds us that we do not simply respond to bodies, we respond to people, negatively or positively. This has profound implications for the regimes of institutions which care for old people, or indeed others needing a high level of physical care, as well as for all who provide such care in the community. Deep feelings are aroused by such activities in those who care, even though these are sometimes personally repressed or professionally suppressed. If these are disregarded by those who employ or are involved with carers, the people being tended are made more vulnerable to exploitation or even abuse. Impersonal physical care is a contradiction in terms. The way we touch, lift and support and the words which accompany actions all convey feelings to the person concerned: they may be experienced as hating or as loving even when the carer disclaims involvement. Indifference is not neutrality, and even in a controlled professional relationship the quality of physical care is emotionally significant.

In an essay on personality, Ungerson (1983a) makes the following comment:

> The central sphere for the operation of the passions is the reality of face to face relationships. The more continuous and lasting a direct interpersonal encounter, the harder will it be for the encounter to assume a purely instrumental quality.

This means that we must acknowledge the powerful emotional expressive components even in interpersonal transactions of an apparently impersonal kind. (The implications for paid staff are further considered in Chapter 7.) Tending, therefore, involves a transaction between carer and cared for, which has powerful emotional undertones, varying in kind and in intensity, but which are always present and affect the way physical care is offered. The extreme vulnerability of frail old people leaves them open to abuse if such matters are not recognised by those who manage services or support carers.

The low status accorded to the work cannot be divorced from the fact that so many of those who provide tending services are women. The extent to which this need remain so tightly gender-related is debatable. A sizeable number of old and younger men provide such care for their own elderly relatives and, in our generation, we have seen some men assume 'mothering' tasks for their children to a greater degree than in the past. Yet the shift is perceived by many as marginal. Ungerson (1983b) discusses 'why do women care?' and raises many important questions.

> We remain ignorant as to the basis of this consistent and apparently universal outcome (that wives and mothers spend a great deal more time tending than their husbands). Is this . . . the result of explicit and implicit discussions made with families? . . . On what basis are these decisions being made? Do they derive from the power of men over women in the domestic arena and/or the labour market, or do they reflect the wishes of the carers themselves, or the assumptions about sex roles embedded in social policies or the ideology of sex-role stereotyping and prevailing ideas of women's proper place . . .

She points out that we know little of the differential impact of changing material circumstances on different kinds of tending, and is surely right when she argues that it would be 'useful and interesting to discover how long term unemployment alters conjugal roles as far as caring is concerned'. So far as I am aware, we have no evidence, for example, to show whether male unemployment which in some areas has been higher than the rate for females, has enabled tending tasks of old relatives to be taken on by men who remain at home.

However, that there is nothing inherently unacceptable in the idea of males performing tending tasks is shown by the established presence of men in nursing and of the increasing numbers employed as care assistants, even in domiciliary care. The extent to which, in informal care, it is acceptable for men to care for women in relation to more intimate tasks is variable and seems that gender taboos are less likely to apply when a man is caring for his wife, than, say, a son for his mother. In professional relationships, gender taboos are weaker.

The combination of changing employment patterns with the increase of numbers of frail elderly people in society, make it appear highly desirable that there should be greater flexibility in the roles allocated to men and women, in relation to domestic arrangements and external employment. Feminists may, understandably, deplore a likely consequence of male intrusion into this woman's world – wages will improve and men may take jobs hitherto only wanted by women! This will be a price worth paying only if the vital expressive quality of the work is sustained and enhanced; that is to say, whether the carer be man or woman, the tasks to be performed involve a relationship with the old person and one in which the essential core of the response should be benign and experienced by the old person as loving. That is an immensely difficult and important goal, which demands preservation of, and respect for, those qualities involved in tending which have been traditionally attributed to femininity, whether they repose in men or women.

CHAPTER 5

Care in the community III: The formal sector

It is not realistic or helpful to view the two sectors, of formal and informal care, as separate. Indeed, the way in which they interact is of crucial importance. However, it is time to focus upon important issues which are centre stage for those who work in the formal sector.

Although the phrase 'care workers' is not in general use, the term has been chosen to describe a wide range of people who may be employed in the voluntary or statutory sectors and who have responsibility for the services made available in the community to support old people and their caring relatives. Any commentary must acknowledge at the outset the difficulty in effectively representing diversity of both sectors in terms of quality, quantity and of 'style', that is to say, in the attitudes and values that underpin service. In such a small country as the United Kingdom, there are striking variations, impossible to explain or justify in terms of need. This point has been made strongly about the Home Help Service, arguably the most crucial support for old people in the community, by Goldberg and Connelly (1982), and more recently by the Audit Commission (1985). It is apparent that not only do actual levels of expenditure per head of the elderly population vary greatly between local authorities, but there are also striking differences in the way the money is spent, for example in the level of support provided to the heavily dependent compared with that for the less dependent. But this only exemplifies a much more general unevenness in such welfare provision, affected by many external factors such as local authority politics.

Nor is such variation in any way particular to the local authority element in the statutory sector. An example from the Health Service, of especial importance to frail elderly people, is in the area of general practice; the entrenched pattern of independent salaried practitioners has resulted in marked differences in standards of professional care which many have argued are unacceptably great. There is no obligation on general practitioners to keep age/sex registers of their patients, a device which lays the foundation for more effective preventive health care of elderly people.

In the voluntary sector, the diversity is even more striking. However, the freedom to provide or not to provide is regarded as an essential element in that sector, and therefore does not attract the same critical comment. From the point of view of those who plan services, however, differences in the overall quality and mix of the elements is bewildering. For example, one of the best known voluntary organisations, Age Concern England, is in fact a federation of local groups. As a federation the centre has no control over (though considerable influence on) the local groups, who are free to develop services however they wish. Indeed, various areas may have no such groups. As a consequence, the local Age Concern Groups differ markedly in what they provide and how they provide it. In particular, they vary in the extent of their involvement with the very frail and housebound, some preferring to concentrate on provision for younger elderly people.

It is nonetheless clear that many valuable inititatives in the care of frail elderly people have arisen from the voluntary sector and few would seriously dispute a model of partnership between voluntary and statutory endeavour. The former may well be of crucial importance in relation to ethnic minorities in the next decade, as the numbers of the very old in these groups increases. So far, a good deal of the efforts of such organisations have been understandably directed to the 'young' old, for example, in providing recreational and cultural facilities for Asians or Afro-Caribbeans. As the numbers grow, it is to be hoped that the voluntary organisations will be pivotal in local planning for the specific needs of the very old in these minorities, both in terms of actual provision and also by drawing the attention of the statutory services to particular needs and problems.

Many would argue fiercely for local autonomy, in both sectors, which makes it possible to develop flexibly and to take responsibility at a local level. There are certainly powerful arguments against centralised systems of welfare and this would in any case run counter to present trends which urge more effective relationships with informal, very local systems of care. However that may be, we are dealing with a curious amalgam of services which has little coherence or consistency. Conventional wisdom, such as the belief that innovation and experiment is the prerogative of the voluntary sector rather than the statutory, is simply not borne out in practice. Such experiments pop up here and there, in both sectors. For example, a local Age Concern group in one area ran a highly imaginative scheme of 'respite care', in which the Manpower Services Commission community programme was used to provide workers to go into carers' homes to provide relief. In other parts of the country, social service departments have developed schemes for intensive domiciliary care to support the old who are alone, with similarly impressive benefits.

The nature of the relationship between the two sectors is also extremely variable at local level. This is partly related to political values; traditionally, organised voluntary activity has been viewed with greater favour by those on the political right, although in fact, unobtrusively, voluntary organisations have received much support by the old-style left. More recently, the emergence of a more radical left wing element in local politics increased tension with the voluntary sector, as, for example, in Liverpool. Nearly all voluntary organisations depend to a substantial extent on funding from statutory services. This has major implications for the relationship between the two; few local 'voluntaries' can afford to offend those who hold purse strings and the nature of the services which they offer may sometimes be on the basis of a contract from the statutory sector (for example, for meals-on-wheels) rather than an independent initiative. It is fair to add, however, that voluntary initiatives do emerge and prosper, sometimes financed, wholly or in part, by the statutory sector.

We have concentrated thus far on the two sectors statutory and voluntary, by which most formal care in the community is delivered. However, in reality the picture is more complicated. The private sector also plays a part, and may do so increasingly, notably in the provision of private domiciliary care. The arrangements which people make privately for various domestic services are well known and little questioned, although practitioners need to be aware of them and relate to the people concerned in planning packages of care. Recently, however, we have seen a growth in the number of private registered agencies, some of which set out to provide a combination of domestic and personal help to frail elderly people. The field has been well surveyed by Midwinter (1986). He points out that although the overall significance of the trend may be exaggerated, 'it is very striking and telling in character'. A characteristic which he stresses, and which should give managers in the formal sector pause for thought, is its 'enormous flexibility'.

> Gardening, house maintenance; holiday sitting or travelling companions; outside window cleaning; help with house moves; small repairs inside and out; decorating; plumbing; electrical work; carpet and upholstery cleaning; pet and plant care.

More needs to be known about the operation of such agencies before one can judge whether the advantages of such flexibility are offset by disadvantages. For example, it would be interesting to know how far they would be prepared to deliver service to frail old people who present particular problems, if they can make a living with easier clients. Furthermore, the quality of staff, as always, is critical and much would depend on their pay and conditions of service.

Encouragement of the private sector could take the form of providing 'cash' (perhaps in the form of tokens or vouchers) by which old people, without adequate financial support, could purchase the services which they require.

This, it may be argued, would increase choice and independence for elderly people. Since many such private arrangements work well now for those with the means, it is clearly inconsistent to resist their expansion without careful thought. The central problem would seem to be market vagaries; old people should not be denied the services which they need to survive in the community because there happens to be a shortage in a given locality, or because certain areas are not profitable, or because some old people are less congenial than others. Furthermore, the stigmatising effects of a residual model of service provision, by which the state intervened with direct help only when all else fails, would be of great concern.

Midwinter does not restrict his discussion of domestic help to private house-holders. The implications go wider and include additional inputs to sheltered housing and the provision of meals. As with private residential care, feelings tend to run high about these trends and are bound up with personal and political preference. However, whatever balance between sectors one would like to see as the basis for community care policy, the private sector is here to stay and likely to expand. It is therefore important that practitioners take cognisance of its existence in relation to the needs of elderly people. It must also surely be important for local government to consider its role in relation to such provision. As Midwinter suggests:

> It should be the collective role of the local authority social services depart-
> ments to have oversight of all who need domiciliary care. Where private
> care is offered by private employment agencies, central control is already
> being exerted under the Employment Agencies Act but local authorities
> do need to monitor the performance of whatever scheme is being operated
> and ensure that gaps in provision are identified and filled.

In matters of this kind, in which support at home to frail elderly people is critical, there is a powerful argument for local government to assume overall responsibility for strategic planning in addition to providing service. This would be to ensure that, through the vagaries of voluntary or private developments, some old people are not left stranded. At present, however, the exact nature of the statutory responsibility is vague and outdated. The Health Services and Public Health Act 1968 empowers a local authority to promote the welfare of old people. Greengross (1986) suggests, that using this as a basis, there should be a general power

> which would enable local authorities to formulate a comprehensive
> policy for the promotion of the welfare of elderly people in their area.

Greengross proposes a *power* rather a *duty* and adds that 'there would be no unreasonable intrusion'. (She suggests, however, that a local authority should have a duty 'to consider the case of a vulnerable elderly person' who may need protection, see Chapter 2.) Whilst accepting the need not to impose more general duties on local authorities when there are severe resource constraints, it may be that some greater legal specificity is required. At present it is only home helps which local authorities have a duty to provide. The degree of priority which social service departments accord to different groups is affected, *inter alia*, by statutory duties and there is always a danger that the needs of the very old people will be neglected in favour of those such as children and families where statutory obligations are more clear cut.

Social ambivalence towards old people plays a part in these somewhat muddled expectations from those who care for them. Although it was not always so, the role of the state in the protection of children is now firmly established. In consequence, when children die from neglect or are maltreated by their carers, questions are always asked about the role of the formal carers; implicitly or explicitly, there is an assumption that formal care systems have in some way been deficient. Hence the numerous child abuse inquiries which have scrutinised, in minute detail, the actions of the professionals involved.

The protection of children has been the subject of important detailed legislation and much guidance from central government. In contrast, the state has played little role in the protection of women against domestic violence although a very active voluntary sector has developed in the past 20 years. Nor does the state assume unequivocal responsibility for old people's well-being. There is no clear professional accountability when tragedies occur although there are some signs of it emerging. When an old person dies alone and is not found until weeks later, 'where were the social services?' is the question sometimes asked by the coroner and the media. But the question is not pursued with the same tenacity and intensity as when a child dies in tragic circumstances. There are two interlocking reasons for this.

Firstly, as we have earlier shown, old people are not valued in the same way as children; their suffering does not pull at the public heart-strings so strongly.

The second, and more positive, factor which may explain the fact that accountability for tragic death is not so readily attributed to the professionals concerns the status of old people as autonomous adults. The concern of civil libertarians, that we should not do things *to* or *about* old people which run counter to their wishes, is entirely legitimate. Their right, as adults, to choose their own life-style, is clearly a principle which should be vigorously upheld. In practice, this may mean that old people are exposed to risk in their own homes and that there will be, on occasion, tragic consequences. It is therefore possible to argue that an analogy with child protection is misleading, since we do not assume that children should look after themselves. It is easy, however, for rhetoric about freedom and choice to blur the reality which professional workers encounter daily. Of the very old, about one in four will have a substantial degree of mental infirmity, often dementia, which seriously impairs their capacity to function competently in a domestic setting. Many others, though not mentally impaired, are very seriously disabled physically. For such old people one has to ask whether acceptance of their professed wish to stay at home carries with it a responsibility to protect them from the consequences of their infirmity. The answer appears to be 'yes, up to a point'; for much of our service provision is focused on support of such people, yet it is patently inadequate in so many ways. This is not, as some cynics might suggest, simply because the alternatives of residential care are in such short supply and such an expensive resource. Most formal carers want to allow old people to remain in their homes as long as possible. This is associated with an acceptance of a duty to support. Yet, as we have seen, the legislative basis of this is, to say the least, vague.

Thus we can see that an uncertainty exists about formal support for old people in the community which contrasts oddly with the general acceptance of accountability for those in residential care, even in the private sector. To ignore those who live at home is unacceptable; it runs counter to a general sense of social responsibility. Yet to take those responsibilities seriously has huge resource implications which would make any government wary of enunciating them in legislation of a more comprehensive and precise kind than currently exists. As the numbers of frail old people grow, in both absolute and proportional terms (and they far exceed any other vulnerable groups), those who work with and for them are bound to experience this dilemma more acutely, which may be summarised as 'just how much are we supposed to do to support and protect such old vulnerable people?'.

At the present time, although certain services, such as those of the family practitioner, are used quite widely by old people over 75, the personal social services are still relatively little used. Only about 13 per cent receive social services in one form or another; about 2 per cent see a social worker. Even though these figures increase quite sharply for old people over 75, it is still a minority of that population. We have little idea of how well other old people cope without the help of the formal sector, though it is not unreasonable to suppose that many struggle in a considerable degree of discomfort and risk. Thus, even if we assume that a significant proportion are well supported either by relatives or by services purchased with their own money, it is highly probable that personal social services see only the tip of an iceberg of unmet needs. Workers know this intuitively from their daily experience and this adds to their strain.

The dilemma for the formal carer is further compounded by a variation on the old theme – 'who is my client?'. Old people do not live in a social vacuum, pursuing their personal goals in ways which do not impinge on others. There is a cost to others incurred by the old person's decision to stay at home. The 'others' may be neighbours, relatives or friends. There may come a point when the rights and needs of other people have to be taken into account in the planning which is done for old people and it is morally unacceptable to take a stance which disregards others' interests. For example, this sometimes arises when an old person who is demented turns night into day, and persistently interrupts the sleep of neighbours, or when his or her home has become so unhygienic it threatens the health and well-being of others. Such behaviour and its effects may rightly affect decisions as to where they should live. For the sake of relatives, decisions may have to be made which are apparently unwelcome to the old person. Leaving aside the obvious example of admission to residential care, there are many less significant matters in which, for example, the old person's attachment to the primary carer makes them reluctant to let anyone else play a part in their support. To ignore the interests of relatives is neither ethically justifiable nor practically helpful if we wish to involve them in care.

Behind the daily activities of those engaged in such formal community care lie stressful moral and practical dilemmas. They are concerned with what is perceived to be 'right' for individual old people and their supporters and what degree of professional responsibility and organisational accountability the workers have for such people.

Individually, workers may feel that they are severely limited, even powerless, in what they can do. But as agents of formal caring systems, they do in fact hold a great deal of power which can be exercised as much by withholding as by giving. One has only to think of the range of services to which an old person may or may not be entitled to see that, even if power is in general exercised responsibly, old people and their informal carers are particularly vulnerable to professional neglect, abuse of power or, more often and more excusably, to inexpert or biased assessment. Virtually all the services which old people need are allocated through formal channels, whether it is home helps, day care, aids and adaptations, or the time of a remedial therapist. The availability of such services plays a part in whether an old person is able to stay at home. Just as a doctor may decide to switch off a life support machine because the patient is in effect dead, so care workers could 'switch off' the services on which the old person is totally dependent for care in the community, thus making admission to an institution inevitable. The fact that this rarely happens (or, where it does, we are not told), reveals the moral repugnance which we would feel at such coercive action. Yet it illustrates vividly the extent of the power which may be implicit in the relationship between care worker and old person. Given the fact that many of the old people concerned are of a generation, class and gender that has traditionally been deferential, it is small wonder if they are characteristically timid and grateful in these exchanges! The 'awkward' minority, Norman (1980) points out, may all too readily be labelled as mentally infirm, despite their right to be 'sad, bad tempered, unsociable or eccentric', like anyone else.

Care in the community is not a kind of moral absolute which should be preserved whatever the costs. We need to examine the case for it in relation to each and every old person, whose circumstances vary so greatly. What then goes into the making of the case? There are four main factors:

1. the wishes and feelings of the old person;
2. the extent and nature of the support needed;

3. the extent and nature of the support available;
4. the extent and nature of the risks attached to it.

The wishes and feelings of the old person are properly our first consideration, though, even if there is no risk to others, one cannot necessarily in all circumstances make them paramount. This is illustrated by the case of the old person who wishes to go into residential care, who is fit and well but wants the comfort and security which it is considered such care will provide. At present, such an old person, if assessed for statutory care, will in all probability be rejected as too fit. (It is interesting that residents of voluntary homes are younger and fitter on admission than those entering statutory or private care. It seems that there are some for whom this is a preferred option, especially when homes have some specific religious or social affiliation.) Private homes increasingly provide another avenue for such old people because of the availability of social security payments without functional assessment for those eligible. If some form of assessment of need for such care is introduced, as seems likely, we shall then have a situation in which old people with private means can choose such care but most will have to prove need. Is it right that there should be two classes of old people in this important respect? Yet, is it right that an old person should be able to enter residential care to be supported by the state regardless of his or her physical or mental state?

Such dilemmas show how these issues and decisions – and the stance which we take on them – are shot through with value judgements about what is 'best' and 'justifiable'. Similarly, when we turn to care at home, it is not clear that if the costs of such support were to exceed those of residential care, they could or should be met. There will also be a limit on the rights of the old person to stay there if the costs, in social and emotional terms, are too high for others. However, some feel that these costs are now too high too often and that the breakdown of a carer, which then precipitates admission to care, is a tragic price to pay for such a choice on the part of the old person. It is further argued that, in the case of those who are mentally frail, they may no longer be capable of exercising informal consent or its converse – refusal; and that resistance to leaving their own home may sometimes be as much about fear of the unknown as love of the familiar. These are all substantial and serious points which make specific decisions for and with individual old people morally onerous and professionally demanding.

The extent and nature of the support which is necessary and available will obviously affect the way in which the situation is appraised. In recent years, we have become more sensitive to the complications which this involves, and the ways in which the formal and informal networks interrelate in successful support systems. It has become fashionable to talk of 'packages' of care. Such packages, when opened, are found to contain many different ingredients of different size and weight which together make it possible for life to be lived at home with a tolerable degree of safety and comfort. The term does not convey the extent to which the different elements in the package depend on each other for the viability of the whole.

It is for this reason that a study carried out by Addison (1984) in the London Borough of Wandsworth, of the social care plans that were made for just two elderly people is of such value, and worthy of attention from practitioners in this field. Addison studies the packages under the following heads:

1. inputs of time, i.e. the length of overall contact, the frequency and regularity of visits and their overall duration;
2. their make-up, i.e. formal and informal networks;
3. key workers and coordination of the packages;
4. the use of meetings in the process.

She analyses such factors as the use of donated time, i.e. time given 'over the odds', and the nature of formal and informal networks which supported the two old people. These networks were extensive, varied and overlapping. They 'did not remain static but became more extensive and complex over time'. They contained 'a range of people with distinctive skills, contributions and perceptions'. Both formal and informal networks tended to divide into sub-networks and problems arose when these were not brought closely together. Especially problematic was the fact that the informal and formal networks never came together nor were the views and opinions of the informal network adequately appraised by the formal care givers who had the responsibility for overall coordination. Support systems which form a package are complex and dynamic. This appraisal requires a kind of mental moving map. A weekly flow chart, showing day by day and hour by hour, who and what is coming into an old person's home to provide care, is useful in illustrating the reality of community care.

In one way and another, and with varying degrees of proficiency, social and health care workers across the country are constructing such packages of care. One particular experience, which has attracted much attention, has been systematically evaluated and has been replicated, through the work of the Kent University Personal Social Services Research Unit. The unique feature is that social workers were given authority to spend up to two-thirds of the cost of a place in residential care in order to support an old person in his or her own home, who would otherwise require such a place. This interesting scheme has been described in detail by Challis and Davies (1987) and appears to have been successful on economic, social and psychological measures. One of the unanswered questions is why, given its declared success, it has not been more widely adopted by local authorities? To understand that would be to throw important light on the relationship between researchers and policy makers.

So what of risk? The term is used to cover different types of situation but in practice it usually refers to the danger to old people's health and safety which may arise when they live alone and are very frail, either physically, mentally or both. The domestic environment is full of hazards, as every mother of young children knows, and it needs a similarly practised eye to spot the potential dangers for old people. However, living is a risky business! No good parent denies children the right to risk themselves physically, socially and emotionally as part of their development and this continues in adult life. For old people living alone or together, there will be risks which they and others may feel is a price worth paying for a richer and more fulfilling life. It is, however, unfortunate that many old people are at risk of injury because of the home circumstances in which they live; some of these hazards could relatively easily be removed. This is of concern because accidents in old age are often permanently disabling and create precisely the dependence which the old person has wished to avoid. The fractured hip so characteristic in frail old women is not infrequently caused by falls at home and these are often occasioned by trivial and remediable household problems – the frayed stair carpet, the trailing flex and so on. The misery to the old person is considerable as is the expense to the National Health Service. Local programmes to help old people view their homes from the point of view of accident prevention and to provide assistance in remedying problems could form a vital part of a preventive strategy which would tackle a commonplace but nonetheless highly significant element in the risks of community care.

Steps are often taken to minimise risk where mental infirmity makes old people unreliable in their behaviour. Hazards associated with heating and walking are examples of matters to which care workers must attend. As with so much work with old people, it is attention to detail which counts: it may make the difference between safety and danger, just as it will between comfort and discomfort. However, the difficulties of containing risk go far beyond the immediate physical environment; they relate also to old people's capacity for self-care, keeping themselves clean, feeding themselves and so on. It is here that some of the thorniest decisions arise about choice and independence. What is the point at which care workers, as agents of society, reject the right of the old person to stay as they are? Clearly, that point is reached if the conditions in the old person's household are a danger to others or cause grave offence. But even if that does not arise, it is unreasonable to expect care workers to accept without anxious questioning standards which fall far below those normally required. Indeed, extensive neglect is likely to be a reflection of mental infirmity of one kind or another. It is, after all, a basic instinct to keep oneself clean and to eat. It is possible that those who theorise about choice and independence are sometimes out of touch with the misery and squalor in which a small number of old people live. However, it is important to acknowledge that judgements about old people's living conditions and standards are, inevitably, coloured by the background and attitudes of the care workers. While there may be agreement about the lowest levels, below which standards cannot be allowed to fall without grave risk to the old person and probably others, individual workers may have very different views and opinions about the acceptability of certain degrees of domestic and personal neglect. This, therefore, plays a part in the differences which sometimes arise in agreeing a plan to support – or not to support – the old person in the community.

Such risk assessment is sometimes complicated by the pressure from relatives who do not live near. They may become very anxious about the risk to which the old person is exposed and urge admission to residential care. In such a situation, it may be that the anxiety springs from not being able to offer more support. One should not be dismissive of these feelings. A caring relative who has a strong attachment to the old person may find the vulnerability of the loved one nearly intolerable. They may have a strong urge to provide care which they cannot translate into reality, and they may be acutely uneasy as a result. They may have mental pictures of disaster which are profoundly disturbing. We should not too readily assume that this is a product of guilty conscience, as a result of deliberate rejection of responsibility, although that may sometimes account for the pressure brought on formal carers to find a solution more comfortable to the complainant. Pressure from relatives can reinforce the worker's anxiety. To fasten one's emotional seat-belt is not easy but the first consideration – that of the old person's needs and wishes – has to be kept constantly in mind.

Another source of anxiety about risk comes from other professionals and has complex origins. There may be genuine differences of opinion about the desirability of continuing community care for that person. Sometimes this is attributable to ignorance of the real alternatives available to the old person, sometimes to different value positions as to what is important – comfort *versus* independence, for example. Another factor may be the time taken in coping with a particular old person which is seen as disproportionate in relation to other work which has to be done.

These and other factors are frequently present in other high risk situations such as child abuse. In such cases, as in the community care of frail elderly, the involvement of different professionals in working together makes it inevitable that such differences of perspective and emphasis will arise. Cooperative activity is central to effective community work and it is therefore to these matters that we turn in concluding this chapter.

One of the persistent misconceptions about professional work in the human service occupations is that it mainly takes place face to face with clients or patients and that time spent with others about the client or patient is a necessary but regrettable adjunct to the real work. Obviously the ratio of direct to indirect work varies with different occupations but, in nearly all, practitioners find that they spend more time on the latter than they think is appropriate. This suggests that something is amiss with the job definition and, by implication, also with education and training which does not prepare them for the reality. In no field is this more obvious than in community care of frail elderly people, for the coordination of services, some from different agencies, is pivotal to their well-being. The fact is that all developed societies undergo processes in which professions and occupations proliferate and become more specialised and we then have to evolve means of 'getting it all together again', in this case, ensuring that the patient or client does not suffer as a result of our separate functions and roles. This, it is suggested, is an inescapable responsibility in community care and is central, rather than tangential, to most practitioners' work.

Community care poses particular problems for such activity. Superficial references to team work gloss over the fact that most of those who are required to act cooperatively are not members of a team in the usual sense. To contrast that group with a hospital team is to see that clearly. They come together much less frequently, from distinct and different settings, and they know much less about each other than do the members of a hospital team, who gain a natural and unforced understanding of each other's roles and characteristics, and adapt accordingly.

Cooperative activity is essential, yet difficult to develop and sustain. Further understanding of the processes involved must be developed. If we take it seriously, we will want to learn more about a range of factors which affect it.

There are four key factors which illustrate the point. Firstly, the effect of attitudes towards, and values concerning, frail elderly people and their carers is critical. Earlier chapters of this book make it clear that there are certain to be tensions, even conflict, on such matters between those who work together. There may be unacceptable ageism in some, negative attitudes towards carers in others. There may be sincerely held differences concerning the level of acceptable risk. Unless these matters are faced, there is a hidden iceberg which threatens the good ship cooperation.

Secondly, one has to understand the effects of the relative status and perceived power of the parties. We note especially the deeply entrenched hierarchical roles in the health professions, the potential for conflict between health and social services personnel, who each control key resources which the other needs, and the effects of gender on individual interactions.

Thirdly, there is a need for better appreciation of the complex dynamics which are at work in small task-focused groups, such as those which come together for case conferences, especially when anxiety about an individual old person is running high.

Fourthly, reference has already been made to the need for cooperation to be perceived as beneficial. At field level, this implies a sufficient understanding of the contribution which different parties can make. It is also affected by the attitudes of those in the respective management structures, who have power to reward in specific ways the activities of their subordinates. Are there 'brownie points' for cooperation?

In short, structural changes alone will not adequately raise the level of cooperative activity. Individuals are profoundly affected by their occupational socialisation, through training and through day-to-day work. The greater the distance, social, geographical and occupational, between those who are supposed to work together, the more likely it is that unhelpful stereotypes will flourish and that there will be fundamental misconceptions about others' roles and functions. In the interests of old people, attention must be paid to these matters.

Another significant area for cooperation lies in the relationship between the formal and the informal sectors whose interactions are usually of primary importance in the support of old people. Reference was earlier made to work of Abrams (in Bulmer, 1986) whose findings and commentary on this issue are equally illuminating. Abrams argues that traditional, local social networks of social care – except as a system of care between kin – are irretrievably lost, but that the new form of 'neighbourhoodism' is a potential or actual substitute, found in 'the formal projects and schemes of the new neighbourhoods'. 'Their emergence and effectiveness', however, are 'tied to the fact that they are making demands. This in turn means that instead of patronising or colonising the community, existing statutory and voluntary agencies are going to have to live with it as an equal'. In practical terms, this creates a different and exciting aspect of work for care workers who may seek to engage constructively with a wide variety of neighbourhood care schemes. However, old people who need help do not initiate such schemes. Sometimes the people engaged in them will have attitudes to, and feelings about, old people which are not acceptable and may even be ageist. Practitioners therefore have an important role in social education.

When one attempts to describe and discuss this elusive concept of community care, one is immediately beset by the range and variety of the situations in which old people find themselves, and of the provision which is made by formal and informal carers in different areas. When one adds to that the immense variation in the capacities and abilities of the old people concerned, the possibility of making valid generalisations seems remote. For workers at field level, a first and necessary step is to make a kind of local map, in which they seek to pinpoint the characteristics of the neighbourhoods which they serve and what is currently available which can be built upon. This is an *environmental assessment* which complements the assessments made of individual old people and their immediate domestic context. Such a procedure will provide important background information for the making of plans for individuals. If the relationship between formal and informal sectors is purposeful and dynamic, these 'maps' will be rather untidy and always changing. Indeed, it may not always be easy for workers in the formal sector to tolerate the muddle and uncertainty which sometimes surrounds informal care activity. The extent of such informal activity will vary greatly in different areas and the extent to which it can be stimulated is unclear. Furthermore, it is the responsibility of formal carers to ensure that the least attractive and approachable of the old people, if they need help, are not neglected by informal care systems or, if that is unavoidable, that they are helped in other ways.

The role of formal carers is a challenging one, full of difficulties but also of opportunities to build services, systems and structures which support very old people in their own homes. The nature of the task requires cooperative activity of a high order at various levels and between a wide range of people. As the Audit Commission (1986) so cogently pointed out, the structural divisions between the health, housing and personal social services have created formidable barriers to cooperation. The Griffiths report (Griffiths, 1988) has recently reviewed community care policy, and we await the government's discussions on its recommendations for financial and structural arrangements. However, it can be confidently predicted that no organisational change will lessen the need for improved interprofessional and interpersonal interactions in the provision of formal care. Structural change may, however, facilitate such interactions.

CHAPTER 6

The practice of assessing elders

Michael Key

This chapter examines issues of assessment confronted by practitioners in different settings. It reviews current practices and offers suggestions for their improvement through the development of affirmative assessment.

Improving the practice of assessing elders is one of the challenges facing practitioners today. This is not just because of the enormous scale of the demands which an ageing population puts on caring organisations. It is also because improving practice in the area of assessment can be done without requiring large increases in financial resources. For these reasons it is worth considering carefully the kinds of approach to assessment that are currently available, and examining ways of improving these.

One traditional approach to assessment is stereotypical labelling by practitioners. Sometimes this appears as a 'pen portrait' of an elder in which moral judgements rather than evaluation predominate. More sophisticated variations may inappropriately use concepts drawn from such disciplines as medicine and psychology, describing elders as 'confused', 'demented', or 'introverted' without adequate evidence. Such an approach can bring the whole notion of assessment into disrepute, as well as misunderstand particular individuals.

This approach to assessment is in decline, although unfortunately not yet extinct. It is being replaced by two newer sorts of approach. Both approaches remedy some of the worst features of labelling, and therefore can be welcomed as advances in practice. Neither, however, are adequate for generating a full picture of elders, and more work is needed to achieve this. The first of these current approaches is that of *functional assessment*.

Functional assessment

This approach moves away from the personal judgements of care givers towards an objective description of the present capacity of an elder to perform in certain physical, psychological and social ways. Sufficiency of performance is taken to mean that an elder can function as an ordinary person without requiring extra support. Conversely, the assessment of insufficient performance points clearly to the sort of services necessary to redress or compensate for functional deficits.

Functional assessment appears to have developed to avoid the limitations of other traditions of diagnosis. For example, Fillenbaum (1985) observes that medical diagnosis 'does not adequately identify people with similar needs for care'. The strength of functional assessment is to point out that an elder who cannot dress will require the same care, irrespective of whether this condition results from a stroke, severe arthritis, an obsessional neurosis, or a low self-esteem. Since the care will be the same, it is not crucial to examine historical causes.

Fillenbaum indicates that the main *areas* of functional assessment chosen for operational use are activities of daily living, physical and mental health, social life, and economic status. The *focus* of such assessment has already been noted as that of current, rather than past or future, level of functioning. The main *methods* are the use of instruments such as checklists, rating scales and questionnaires. These ensure systematic assessment, and can be tested for reliability and validity. These methods give functional approaches an affinity with the selective approach to assessment that will be considered later. The main *uses* of functional assessment seem to be to select from available services to remedy any incapacities assessed, to help to prevent functional deterioration, and to highlight areas of functioning which merit fuller assessment than can be achieved by this approach.

A number of instruments have been developed to measure the functioning of elders. CAPE tests (Pattie and Gilleard, 1979) may be familiar to many British practitioners. Those wishing to examine such instruments are directed to Fillenbaum (1985), Kane and Kane (1981), and Woods and Britton (1985), who all give extended reviews of what is available, and to Barrowclough and Fleming (1986) for an application of this approach in goal planning. Although instruments vary in detail, several general limitations can be identified.

Firstly, areas of functional competence are usually derived from the practical concerns of care givers rather than from the viewpoint of elders. Forms of oppression such as sexism and racism, and the effect of the setting in which functioning is assessed, are both too easily ignored. Secondly, instruments tend to dwell on deficits in performance rather than levels of higher competence. Thirdly, the quantitative format of functional assessment lends itself to use by managers and policy makers as survey data instead of as individual assessments. Spurious indicators of difficult concepts such as 'dependency' can result (see for an example Booth (1985)), which can both alter service provision and lead to new forms of labelling.

In normal adult life most of us would feel insulted and demeaned if the basic value we had as human beings was described by the kind of functional assessments that have been discussed. Many practitioners know this, and may be put off from benefiting from the undoubted if limited strengths of functional assessment. Ways of building on these strengths to achieve a more positive approach to assessing elders will be returned to later. First, however, consideration must be given to the other major approach to assessment that informs current practice.

Selective assessment

This second major approach hinges on a distinction that can be made between *selective assessment* and *affirmative assessment*.

Where services are provided on the basis of the principle of universality, such as national insurance retirement pensions, only enough assessment is required to confirm that a person falls within an impersonal category. But where provision is organised on the principle of selectivity, as in the health and personal welfare sectors, more complex assessment is required in order both to ration (or target) resources, and to link correctly an applicant to what is available. In both cases the assessment task can be identified as that of correctly *selecting* individuals, i.e. selective assessment.

Selective assessment is orientated to the interests of the organisation from which the assessment originates. The practitioner works as the officer of the organisation to test for entitlement to its services, perhaps using functional assessment methods. Success typically gives access to one existing service, such as domiciliary care, and rejects another, such as residential care.

In selective assessment the relationship between practitioner and elder is one of unequal power. The practitioner has technical expertise, has some command of the organisation's scarce resources, and is supported by the generalised aura of power that surrounds officials in modern societies. This power imbalance is likely to have a marked effect on the attitudes of elders to sharing information about themselves.

White elders today, and even more so black elders who arrived in the 1950s, belong to a cohort that has often experienced assessment in earlier life as something that selects or rejects. Such assessment is felt to have 'kept people in their places' (i.e. is a method of social control) by testing at school or at work, or through means-tested public and charitable benefits. Although selective assessments may have been endured, practitioners today should anticipate that they will restimulate deep feelings for many who have perceived past treatments as inadequate or unjust. Anxiety, anger or apathy all seem reasonable defensive strategies for elders to adopt when facing selective assessment now.

Yet there are arguable benefits from practising selective assessment. A careful, just and public system of this kind may be a fairer way of deciding between competing bids for scarce resources than leaving the fate of an elder to the personal impressions or abilities of a practitioner. Indeed, equal opportunity policies, and strategies of affirmative action, can be built into selective assessments.

Nevertheless, there are obvious limitations to a system of selective assessment. What is central to the life of an elder may be marginal to each of the several organisations providing services, and, as recently reiterated by the Audit Commission (1986), can easily be missed in their selective assessments. Multidisciplinary and interagency collaboration might avoid this, but at the cost of greater surveillance by the state and commercial bodies. Another weakness is that selective assessment becomes preoccupied with screening for high risk and other needs are ignored. This not only affects individuals, but also slows down service development to meet changing patterns of need. Finally, unless selective assessments are properly evaluated there is no guarantee that they are correctly selecting those for whom existing provision is intended.

Selective assessment cannot be dispensed with while there is a shortage of resources to meet individual needs. It is the public sector alternative to the price mechanism of 'the market' for allocating limited resources – an alternative that has been hotly debated since the origin of the Poor Law. From another standpoint it is impossible, given the infinite unique patterns of need demonstrated by individuals, to provide wholly individualised packages of care provision. Organisations have to provide services in advance of knowing precisely which individuals will use them, and it is inevitable that to some extent the individual has to 'fit in' with what is on offer. Given this, practitioners should neither blindly administer selective assessment procedures, nor dismiss them out of hand. Instead they should become more aware of the strengths and limitations of selective methods, and struggle for more just and refined procedures.

The pursuit of justice can be supported by supplementing selective assessment with *affirmative assessment*. This is focused much more by the perspectives of the elder. Efforts are made to identify an elder's past and current situations, strengths and difficulties, and future potential, all from the elder's point of view. Criteria for doing this are developed from the professional knowledge, value base and experience of the practitioner rather than from the policies and constraints of organisations. Information may be gathered in a variety of ways, including the use of functional assessment instruments and selective assessment forms. The information is used to *affirm* a unique individual profile, from which an individualised plan for the person is developed through a more equal relationship with the elder being assessed. The notion of affirmation thus helps to assert the right of elders to have their unique identities and histories properly acknowledged in any assessment process.

Towards affirmative assessment

Affirmative assessment starts from a basic belief that human beings are purposeful beings who have intentions which guide their behaviour. Elders are not passive objects merely conditioned by stimuli from society or their body. Instead an elder (like any human) is understood as having enough power to act in a way that makes some difference to what happens. An elder's purposes are not simply mental ideals or fantasies, but are working ideas that give direction to daily living.

From this starting point, four theoretical ideas are identified which can contribute to a practice of affirmative assessment. These are the ideas of *consciousness, desire, attachment,* and *suffering.* Although none is fully explored here, all help to understand people better, and they are linked by the belief that we have some control over our destinies.

Consciousness

The idea of *consciousness* is broader than conventional approaches to cognitive functioning which focus on assessing intelligence, memory and language. We have to find ways of assessing general intellectual capacity without resort to the 'silly questions' sometimes used in psychological tests (Woods and Britton, 1985). A more effective approach might be to ask elders about their understanding of their own situation or behaviour in particular places at particular times. Thus, questions about the names of politicians or the days of the week may appear too childish to be taken seriously, whereas discussion of daily activities, and their purposes, may not.

There are three aspects to the idea of consciousness which need to be distinguished (Giddens, 1984). The first is discursive or *verbal consciousness.* This is the ability of a person to talk about his or her actions, reasons for these, and their place in an ongoing flow of social life. This discussion may take several forms, including speech, writing, sign language or even 'talking inside oneself'. For example, an elder may say or write 'I was upset when my wife died, and couldn't get on with doing for myself. I always got on with my daughter, but she's in Canada now, so I asked my son if I could stay with him for a bit. I'd like to move near him, but I'd have to get on the Council list and I don't know if I'd qualify.'

This capacity to analyse feelings, hopes and intentions is taken in our culture as the main criterion for being a 'normal' ordinary adult. Although its development from infancy to early adulthood has been much examined, the part it plays in later life has been largely neglected. This neglect is not only by academics, but is also evident in the practice of both selective and functional assessment. Elders are often denied the status of ordinary adulthood when they are not encouraged to discuss how they see their situation. Elders who sustain high levels of verbal consciousness are unlikely to be perceived as 'old', but rather as continuing 'middle aged' or as having a special status derived from their past education or profession.

Clearly verbal consciousness is related to past learning, and so will vary considerably according to such factors as class, race and gender. Even so, practitioners wishing to avoid ageism should find methods for assessing and recording the competence of an elder to reflect on their situation. Such assessments may help to identify supports which can sustain and enhance this basic capacity of an elder. This aspect of assessment is essential because a person's verbal consciousness is critical for making sense of the world.

However, people do not usually live in a state of high intellectual awareness about their every action, but simply get on with living. The concept of *practical consciousness* is especially helpful in accommodating this commonplace fact. Practical consciousness describes the occasions when a person knows about the situation he or she is in, and how to behave appropriately, but expressess this in actions or perhaps clichéd words. This lies behind the very large number of habitual activities that make up the routines of ordinary day-to-day life. For example, an elder (like the rest of us) will get up, go to the toilet, go through familiar washing routines, make tea, collect the paper from the front door, and perhaps walk down to the shops or catch the bus into town, with competence and efficiency. She or he is 'on automatic', but the ability to perform many such functions is critical for independent life, as functional assessment approaches would recognise.

All this is commonly done without any demonstration of verbal consciousness or deliberate reflection. But practical consciousness can be converted into verbal consciousness in many instances. For example, a neighbour may ask 'what are you doing?' and the elder can say 'I've got to spend a penny, it's these new tablets', or 'I'm going into town for some firelighters'. From such beginnings longer dialogues might result which become increasingly discursive.

This potential to transform practical into verbal consciousness is highly significant if an elder is to be assessed affirmatively, and is easily ignored in functional assessments. Assessing this potential helps the practitioner to decide how best to work with an elder when some breakdown in routine occurs. These include becoming incontinent, being admitted to hospital or residential home, facing changes in the social security system, or being widowed. Any breakdown in routine commonly demands a shift into verbal consciousness while new ways of behaving are learned. In due course, when the transition is successfully achieved, these new ways return to the level of practical consciousness.

Insensitive handling of this process can result from a misassessment of an elder's competence to make these shifts, and of the time and energy this takes. The outcomes of inadequate assessment in this area are evident, for example, in the learned helplessness of institutionalised routines, or the difficulties of transferring skills learned in a rehabilitative setting to a domestic setting.

Successful practice requires a thorough understanding of how a shift from practical to verbal consciousness occurs and may be facilitated. We need to know much more about this, but until these ideas are developed more adequately for use in work with elders, the practitioner may have to be somewhat rough and ready in assessing the capacity of an elder to use both practical and verbal consciousness. This may mean directly asking an elder for an account of her or his behaviour, and, after discussion with the person, forming a provisional judgement. This entails checking the capacity of an elder to receive and send messages. Attention also should be given to facilitating the interaction. For example, an elder's response is likely to be inhibited if the practitioner uses baffling words, or the elder is flustered in a busy doctor's surgery.

From such efforts, different assessments might be made. Firstly, an elder may display verbal consciousness for most of her or his day-to-day conduct, even if sometimes haltingly or with verbal expression impaired by physical conditions such as aphasia. In such cases plans can be made in partnership with an elder, and future intervention can be negotiated with as much (or as little) justice and hope as for any other adult.

Secondly, an elder may display little verbal consciousness at the time of the assessment, but from other information available this may be identified as linked to some crisis, such as bereavement or illness, or a temporary condition such as side-effects of medication. In the short-term, non-verbal approaches to assessment, like the use of functional assessment instruments, will then have to be adopted. But such an elder must be understood as likely to recover verbal consciousness, and should not be assessed as 'confused' or of 'low intelligence'.

Thirdly, some elders may demonstrate little verbal consciousness, but from using functional assessment instruments it seems likely that they are capable of sustaining a largely independent life at the level of practical consciousness. Practitioners could then consider whether this can be transferred to a new physical or social setting, or is sustainable only in a familiar setting.

Fourthly, in some cases elders may be assessed as having little practical consciousness. They no longer function adequately 'on automatic' and may therefore be exposed to unacceptable risks. For example, elders with brain failure may 'make mistakes' (such as not lighting the gas or wandering naked). These are not recognised by the elder as a social error (something possible at the level of practical consciousness) nor as having hazardous consequences (which perhaps requires verbal consciousness).

This aspect of lost practical and discursive consciousness is well recognised in the literature on dementia, although it is usually described in the language of psychogeriatrics. For example Gray and Isaacs (1979) identify such conditions as loss of the mental competence to register new information, of the ability to discriminate between simliar stimuli, of the ability to generalise, and of the ability to relate present events to past experience or future consequences.

Deviant elders should not of course be automatically assessed as confused 'dements'. But where there are irreversible or extensive neurological changes, the assessing practitioner may have to conclude that such an elder has lost the capacity to function independently. Behaviour has become a mechanical outcome of internal physiological and external physical and social forces. In such cases functional assessment methods are indispensable, and show the value of behavioural methods of working that do not assume consciousness as a fundamental human quality. If possible these assessments should be conducted in settings containing opportunities to stimulate the familiar routines of practical consciousness – something unlikely in most interview rooms. As Gray and Isaacs (1979) note, taking an elder with brain failure to a pub can enable that elder to sustain the practical consciousness necessary to have a drink, sing or make a joke.

At first sight it might seem strange to consider *unconscious* forces within a concept of consciousness. However, it is now widely accepted that there are powerful forces of which we are not aware which influence our behaviour. For example, a basic sense of trust about oneself and the world is arguably necessary for a person to function competently. A good deal of this security is located in the routines making up practical consciousness – predictability reduces anxiety. But practitioners usually encounter elders at just those times when crisis has broken down the security of routine. At such times anxiety and other strong emotions of which we are normally unaware can overwhelm, or trigger defences like denial or repression. Such emotional turbulence can produce distress and uncharacteristic behaviour.

For this reason affirmative assessment must go beyond seeing anxiety anger, guilt and sadness as simply newly learned reactions. Yet unconscious processes should not be used by a practitioner as a convenient answer to awkward contradictions. Careful work has to be done with an elder, family and friends in considering the ways in which unconscious elements are affecting current behaviour. One must avoid glib speculations about connections between the past and the present, or between disguised feelings and behaviour. Yet the powerful effect of these hidden forces cannot be denied, and has to be taken into account in assessment. For example, extreme or bizarre reactions to bereavement may have their roots in unconscious feelings belonging to earlier experiences of loss. But although unconscious feelings have traditionally been associated with severe emotional disorder, they are not the prerogative of the acutely disturbed. They colour everyday life, in terms of both verbal and practical consciousness.

The concept of the unconscious has been derived mainly from psycho-analytically based theories and its complexities are beyond the scope of this discussion. Many analysts might argue that the exploration of the unconscious can take place sensibly only within their particular therapeutic discipline, and lies outside the competence of most public sector practitioners. How far such practitioners attempt to facilitate a process in which these less consciously available feelings are related to present attitudes and behaviour must depend, firstly, on their confidence about the validity of such linkages, secondly on their conviction that this is useful, and thirdly on their having the necessary skills. Perhaps the most important point to make is that, as part of affirmatively assessing elders, we should never assume that unconscious processes are less important or less worthy of exploration than they are in other people.

Desire

The concept of need has been widely used in practice and in social policy, and is a complex and confusing one (Bradshaw, 1972). For our purposes it may be more helpful to use the idea of *desire* when assessing elders. We need first to distinguish between *objective requirements* and *subjective desires.*

Objective requirements are the small list of conditions necessary to sustain biological life in an organism. These include certain chemicals and temperatures, but in a laboratory sense which is completely divorced from any cultural meaning. All cultural norms about basic needs for food, shelter and so on are seen by contrast as expressions of subjective desire, even though these desires will have been shaped by the standards of a particular society. In addition to these cultural beliefs about 'basic needs', elders, like everyone else, will display an almost infinite potential to develop other desires for commodities and human experience. Assessing desires is an affirmation of human potential.

Strongly held desires are likely to belong to the level of verbal consciousness. Such desires are easily understood and expressed as conscious wishes – 'I'd really like to be closer to my sister'. Yet it often seems the case that elders have depressed their desires in this category, presenting a picture of low expectations. Such elders may be stoically enduring remediable suffering, have internalised an ageist view that old folks should not have many desires 'at their time of life', or hold a belief that it is wrong to want things, or to be assertive.

The power to assert desires verbally is an essential characteristic of the potent adult. The assessment of such desires – be they feasible or fantastic – gives the practitioner a chance to explore the future potential and development of an elder, and for jointly planning relevant service provision with that person. Giving special attention to exploring such desires with all elders is a hallmark of affirmative assessment. It requires the development of advanced skills in order to overcome communication blocks, whether because of deafness, aphasia, educational background, past work experience, class, race, or gender. Unless this attention is given, practitioners will be unwittingly reinforcing the widespread depressed level of desire found in elderly clients.

Desires experienced at the level of practical consciousness are sometimes hard to assess because they are welded to the objects making up habitual routines. Going to the shops may be done in such an automatic way as to not seem to be the fulfilment of desire at all. Even so, a link between desire and routine behaviour should be noted as an important element in preserving the right of elders to 'want something', and thus to avoid depersonalising them.

Sometimes this link can be explored by careful questioning to convert routines back into verbally expressed desires. More usually such desires can be assessed only speculatively by sharply observing the relationships, beliefs or objects around which routines are focused. This has the further benefit of helping to sustain or extend current routines through various kinds of provision. One must never assume that an elder who cannot discuss personal desires does not need an environment in which such desires can crystallize and find expression.

Some desires in ordinary adults are unconscious. An elder's unconscious may contain a lifetime's thwarted desire in the form of unresolved suffering and pain. This may be contributing to current depression of desire and loss of human potency. Such a state of affairs cannot be ignored, as it tends to be in selective and much functional assessment. It is of importance in its own right, since affirmative assessment aims to include all significant experience, and unconscious pain is surely significant. It is also important to recognise because apparently harmless discussion about 'wants' can restimulate unconscious feelings to the surprise and distress of both elder and practitioner – 'it brings it all back'.

Attachment

Although desires are internal, they are all linked to the external world through objects. In common parlance 'objects' are understood as inanimate 'things'. But in terms of the idea of *attachment* objects can be very varied. As well as animate or inanimate 'things' like people, pets, houses or money, objects can include ideas like self identity, one's beliefs (a religious faith), symbols (the Flag), or relationships (marriage). People can become attached to any or all of these sorts of object.

Whatever the kind of object, it has to be conceptualised in the imagination. For example, an elder saying 'I'd like a nice cup of tea' is clearly linking motivational energy with an imagined object in a way that helps the person to take the action necessary to fulfil the desire. This kind of realistic desire can be distinguished from unrealistic fantasy according to whether or not there is a possible social action which could fulfil the desire. There are also fantasies where there is no serious desire for fulfilment, as in the manner of daydreams. They offer comfort without the need for action.

The works of Bowlby (1979) and Marris (1974) offer the basis for a model of attachment that can be used to assess elders affirmatively. Bowlby suggests a clear cycle of events in which an infant becomes attached to a significant person. This cycle is developed in Table 6.1 in a form applicable for understanding the circumstances of an elder.

An elder will have experienced many attachments to, and losses of, objects of all types. In old age several major losses may occur within a short space of time. Such multiple loss, perhaps taken with earlier experiences of loss, may produce grief that is profound enough to overwhelm the capacity for verbal consciousness. If anguish is too great, an elder may simply cease to discuss loss and just keep going at the level of practical consciousness. In this way basic existential security may be maintained, but at the cost of being less able to desire new attachments to new objects.

For some, perhaps those who have a history of anxiety and many insecure attachments, a diminished capacity to engage in seeking new attachments may represent a welcome relief from endlessly unfulfilled desires. For others in this position it may feel like a forcible disengagement from the quest for security and is regarded with anger or despair. For elders with histories of secure attachments, a diminished capacity to desire new attachments may be accepted sagely as age-appropriate – or feared and rejected as an unwelcome sign of old age and impending death.

These diverse possibilities alert the practitioner to consider sensitive areas of life beyond what can be comprehended through functional assessments of current performance. Not only should an understanding be gained of a history of losses, but also of the potential for new attachments.

Suffering

Some of the effects of loss can be explored by using the idea of *suffering*. Such an idea offers elders, carers and practitioners the opportunity to discriminate between appropriate and inappropriate suffering.

The Oxford English Dictionary definition of suffering – to undergo pain or grief or damage or disablement – implies that suffering is likely to be avoided rather than desired. This fits well with the pain-avoiding hedonistic and utilitarian elements of modern consumerism. Yet even hedonists can value short-term pain as an appropriate means to long-term pleasure, and utilitarians can accept as appropriate individual suffering if its outcome benefits a larger number.

Table 6.1 A cycle of attachment, loss, and reattachment.

1.	No attachment	Anxiety and suffering generate unconscious desires for survival/security which are not met.
2.	Attachment object available	An 'object' which can meet desires and reduce anxieties.
3.	Attachment behaviour demonstrated	High-dependency on physical nearness to the attachment object, and distress (withdrawal or rage) if separated.
4.	Types of attachment achieved	
(a)	*Secure attachment*	Unanxious attachment to the object which externally is equivalent to it becoming the routine of practical consciousness, and which internalises the object symbolically. Reduction of anxiety gives a secure base from which other desires and objects can be explored. Basic trust is secured.
(b)	*Anxious attachment*	Constant anxiety is experienced. There is a low threshold for showing attachment behaviour (e.g., suicide attempt, anorexia, hypochondria) if objects are not available.
(c)	*Compulsive self-reliance*	Ongoing anxiety is repressed by stoic behaviour. There is an inhibition of the desire for objects like close relationships.
(d)	*Compulsive care-giving*	Ongoing anxiety about incomplete attachment to others is converted into compulsive care-giving and the inhibition of own desires.
5.	Loss of attachment object	From temporary or permanent separation.
6.	Types of grief response	
(a)	*Uncomplicated grief*	Movement through recognised stages of grief, some of which include behaviour mirroring attachment behaviour. Typical when previously there was secure attachment.
(b)	*Complicated grief*	Including unusually deep or prolonged feelings of despair, anxiety or guilt, with lengthy depression, suicide or delaying grief. Typical when there were previously insecure attachments.
7.	Appearance of new attachment object	A repetition of step 2.
8.	Further attachment behaviour	A repetition of step 3.
9.	Reattachment	A repetition of step 4.
10.	Further loss of new attachment object	Repetition through the whole cycle.

Other philosophies justify the value of suffering more strongly. Stoicism, like Buddhism, calls for indifference to the material world and a fatalism based on freeing oneself from desires. Without desire there can be no attachment and so no loss and corresponding suffering. Any suffering experienced can be valued as a means of learning about desire and selflessness.

Existential beliefs offer one convenient vehicle to examine some aspects of suffering in a way that links with earlier ideas presented. These beliefs assert that a human existence is composed of all the choices of action (e.g. desires, attachments) made from moment to moment. A person's lifetime experience is understood as the outcome of this permanent struggle to 're-invent' one's being in a universe made up of things, relationships, self and the transpersonal (Van Deurzen-Smith, 1984).

This view of existence assumes that neither pleasure nor pain naturally predominates, but that life is a permanent encounter with both positive and negative elements. These elements may coexist in the same event. Such a framework brings together the contradictions of death, pain, destruction and despair on the one hand, and life, pleasure, creation and joy on the other.

When we make assessments of other people, of any age, and in any capacity, we often have a sense as to whether or not they 'feel real'. In existential theory, this feeling is described by the terms 'authentic' and 'inauthentic'. Most of us are located somewhere on a continuum between these two positions. Being authentic ('feeling real') is bound up with a capacity to accept and live constructively with the contradictions between the positive and negative elements of life. Although aware of the anxieties inherent in seeking attachments, and the risks of loss, an authentic person is likely to be aware of her or his desires to build a meaningful life, and to pursue these with commitment. Being inauthentic ('feeling false') comes from ignoring or denying life's contradictions, perhaps by attaching oneself exclusively to objects which do not involve the sort of deep relationships or beliefs that can give personal pain as well as joy. Extreme preoccupation with the comforts of money, commodities or social status are common examples. Another form of inauthenticity may occur when a person lives largely at the level of practical consciousness, in which routines defend against the anxieties which life itself engenders, and fresh desires are seldom asserted.

When assessing elders affirmatively, the practitioner may well detect in some very old people a remarkable degree of authenticity. Such elders may have given positive meaning to experiences of anxiety, poverty, chronic illness, multiple losses and death. As discussed elsewhere (Key, 1985), it is possible to envisage dying as part of this framework. Certainly hospice experience shows that an elder nearing death who has little functional competence left may demonstrate a degree of human authenticity that indeed makes dying the final stage of growth – 'a good death'. This authenticity seems to incorporate and synthesize suffering, to give a profound and valued richness to a whole life. Such suffering, it is suggested, can be understood as highly appropriate. By contrast, seemingly secure elders may have made inauthentic adaptations to life which are disguised by the routines and objects of daily living. When these adaptations are tested by significant loss, they may be unable to reconstruct a secure world for themselves. This may lead to personal collapse and destructive suffering, as noted by both Marris (1974) and Bettelheim (1970).

Suffering, then, may be appropriate if it can be borne and can contribute towards greater authenticity. In such cases it may need to be supported at the level of verbal consciousness, and, like grieving as the gateway to reattachment, should not be prematurely foreclosed. Yet sometimes such suffering may be too much to bear, and is perhaps best dealt with by an elder attempting to return to former levels of less authentic but endurable adaptations to life. Knowing which kind of support to offer requires the practitioner to use deep empathy based on affirmative assessment.

Existentialism is of course neither the only nor necessarily the best framework in which to locate suffering. It does, however, show clearly that when assessing suffering it is important to have a framework that goes beyond the narrow concerns of selective or functional assessment approaches, although such approaches do have some value in distinguishing between 'appropriate' and 'inappropriate' suffering. Both can satisfactorily detect situations in which inappropriate suffering is occurring because of external deficiencies in food, warmth, income, housing and health. Suffering caused by inefficient distribution of objects (money, services, or goods) is clearly inappropriate.

The appropriateness of suffering during a normal cycle of grief has already been noted. Worden (1983) implies that absence of suffering may be understood as a form of abnormal grief, and in fact may be symptomatic of deeper and unconscious inappropriate suffering – perhaps due to earlier grief reactions. It follows that affirmative assessors must be able to discriminate at least between these two types of grief reaction.

There is another aspect of loss and suffering that cannot be ignored. Some elders may have been obliged to be attached to objects or routines which in some way were exploitative, oppressive or otherwise caused suffering. A changed situation may be welcomed as a release from such suffering, although not without mixed feelings. For example, some who have for years looked after a spouse may sometimes have deeply resented the way that this has taken over their lives, particularly perhaps if this feels forced by cultural assumptions such as 'appropriate' roles for women in the domestic setting. Death of the spouse may give relief from the oppression of selfless caring mixed with guilt about feeling relieved.

It has been suggested that suffering may be appropriate when in some way it contributes to learning and personal growth. Such suffering is a temporary stage in a developmental process. Some suffering is, however, permanently painful, unendurable even, and is neither a transitional stage nor is remediable. Certain chronic or terminal ailments may fit into this category, as may negative aspects of membership of a minority group. This quality of suffering seems to go beyond any classification of appropriateness or inappropriateness. It is mentioned here because encounters with such forms of suffering may distress practitioners so much as to block off their own capacity to deal sensitively and effectively with the people concerned. In this, as in so many matters involving the practitioner in the pain of elders, attention must be given to supporting practitioners so that they can confront their own feelings, fears and anxieties about old age and those whom they seek to help.

This chapter has offered a framework for practitioners to use as they reflect professionally on their practice of assessing elders. As a framework it can make no claim to be exhaustive or final. But it will have been a fruitful exercise if practitioners are themselves encouraged to explore issues of assessment in a more critical way.

CHAPTER 7

Residential care

There is now a substantial literature on the subject of residential care of old people. It deals with broad policy issues, such as the desirable balance between residential and community provision, the dependency levels of people in the homes, and the internal running of the homes. Much of the evidence from research is admirably summarised by Sinclair (1987) and the bibliography in this book cites other useful references for those with a particular interest in the topic. This chapter does not attempt a comprehensive discussion. Rather, it focuses attention on two central and problematic elements in the debate, which tend to arouse strong feelings, both in the general public and in the many different professionals who care for elderly people. These are, firstly, the place of residential care within the wider context of social care provision and, secondly, the difficulties experienced over many years in creating an environment within residential care which preserves the dignity and autonomy of individuals. Most of the discussion centres on care in homes rather than in hospitals but common problems and issues arise in both.

The place of residential care within the wider context of social care provision

Only a small proportion of elderly people live in any form of institutional care, as Table 7.1 shows.

Between 1974 and 1984, there was a slight increase, about 1 per cent, in the numbers of people over 75 living in institutional care. At present about 8 per cent of such elderly people live in homes or hospitals. Very large numbers

Table 7.1   Balance of care for elderly people, England and Wales. (Data from Audit Commission, 1986.)

	1974		1979		1984	
	Number	Number per 1000 over 75	Number	Number per 1000 over 75	Number	Number per 1000 over 75
Occupied hospital beds (geriatrics)	54 600	22.1	54 500	19.6	54 100	17.1
Local authority homes (occupied places)	98 600	40.0	109 100	39.3	109 200	34.5
Nursing homes (long-stay occupied beds)	11 900	4.8	13 800	5.0	24 100	7.6
Voluntary homes (occupied places)	23 300	9.5	25 600	9.2	26 900	8.5
Private homes (occupied places)	19 300	7.8	26 800	9.7	55 000	17.4

of heavily dependent old people are cared for in the community. Table 7.1 reveals significant shifts in the nature of that provision, notably the decline in geriatric beds and local authority provision compared with a rise in private nursing homes and a very steep rise in private rest homes. Local authority residential care is an expensive resource. Elderly people consume 55 per cent of the budget of the personal social services; residential care takes more than half of that budget yet only cares for about 2 per cent of the elderly population. Sinclair (1987) points out that institutional provision for old people in this country is low compared to others. It is argued by some that our level has been too low. A paradox becomes apparent when research findings are analysed. On the one hand, it is clear that most old people say that they would prefer to remain in their own homes. On the other hand, most places in all three sectors are taken up. The rapid growth in the private sector demonstrates that when places become available, they are filled. The probable explanation – and a sad one – lies in the perceived inadequacy of community care support and arrangements and in the attitudes of professionals and relatives to old people. Sinclair concludes his review as follows:

> The vast majority of elderly people do not want to go into residential care. Asked to consider the possibility that they cannot look after themselves at home, most are likely to opt for sheltered housing.

Despite the above, demand for residential care outruns provision and will be increased by demographic trends. Compared to some other European countries England and Wales have few residential places for the elderly: residential beds for the elderly in areas of the country which are generously supplied with them are usually not difficult to fill.

Partly for this reason community care policies have not over the past ten years reduced the numbers in residential care either absolutely or per thousand over 75. Nor has there been a shift of resources in favour of community services for the elderly.

This point has been critically discussed by the Audit Commission (1986) which argues that the growth in private care for which social security payments are available has diverted state resources from community care provision. Nor should we forget that residents who fund themselves in private care (more than half) usually do so out of their one capital asset – their house. In so doing, they are unable to leave to their children a much prized inheritance. While we may differ in the desirability of inherited wealth, it is surely ironic that, during a Conservative administration, there has been a substantial increase in the numbers of old people whose lifetime savings, in the purchase of a house, have to be spent in a manner never envisaged or intended. Nor can the present anomalies concerning charges between the private sector, the local authority and National Health Service be justified. The present picture is one of confusion, of a lack of overarching policies which greatly increases the stress on old people and those who care and plan for them.

Moreover, concern about institutional care of all kinds has been pervasive and longstanding. Several factors in post-war years have led to doubts about the place of institutions in providing care for vulnerable and dependent people, whether they be elderly, mentally handicapped, mentally ill or children.

Firstly, research from the fields of psychology (for example, Barton, 1959) and sociology (for example, Goffman, 1961) demonstrated beyond doubt the adverse effects on the development and behaviour of individuals when they were confined in institutions and subjected to depersonalising regimes. This is not now disputed; argument centres upon the conditions which create these effects and the extent to which they can be remedied.

Secondly, formal research apart, there was a moral revulsion against the basis on which some such care had been provided before the war. Local authority provision, for example, still reminded people of the discredited 'Poor Law' work houses and the incoming post-war Labour government spoke of creating 'hotels' for old people. The Curtis Committee, reporting in 1946 on the plight of children in care, sharply criticised large impersonal institutions. Townsend (1964) strongly attacked much of the local authority residential care for old people on similar grounds. Scandals arose concerning the care of the mentally handicapped in large hospitals. Such studies and enquiries influenced public opinion. In particular, it became clear how difficult it was to modify the regimes of large institutions, especially when they were relatively isolated and caring for people whose dependency resulted in part from degrees of mental infirmity.

Thirdly, increasing emphasis came to be placed upon the principle of 'normalisation'; that is to say, the right of individuals to live a life as nearly as possible similar to others in their society. Whilst those who staff institutions may seek to implement normalisation by providing residents with a life-style as 'ordinary' as possible, there is no doubt that such policies posed particular problems within an institutional context. This contributed to the movement towards community care, as opposed to institutional care.

Fourthly, it became apparent, especially during the 1970s, that institutional care of any kind, for any group, was very expensive. When chill economic winds blew, government took note of the negative view of such care taken by many academics and professionals and, understandably, used such evidence to lend weight to policies of community care, the financial burden of which was, in some degree, less heavy than that of institutions. (How much less depends on the level of community provision.)

While these concerns and criticisms rumbled on, many local authorities sought to minimise the supposed adverse effects of their residential provision by reducing the size of their establishments and by reducing the isolation experienced by residents.

In the field of child care, especially large homes and isolated cottage homes were replaced by smaller 'family group' homes, often placed on local housing estates. Very large old people's homes were replaced by small units, although never as small as those for children – 40-bed homes were the norm. As with children's homes, however, these were often sited in or near ordinary housing. The model of the converted country house, set in spacious grounds, was unacceptable because of the likelihood of isolation.

Size and location, then, were seen as significant factors in creating a residential environment with fewer detrimental effects. It would be cynical not to applaud the efforts made and perverse not to acknowledge that they have played a part in improving the quality of life for residents. Nevertheless, the whole history of residential care shows how difficult it has been to construct an environment which provides the conditions conducive to residents' social and emotional well-being. Various factors play a part in this, some of which are the subject of the second half of this chapter.

In summary, therefore, we have a situation in which small numbers of very old people are cared for at great expense in establishments where most of them would prefer not to be and in which, as will be shown later, it is difficult to offer a satisfactory quality of life. What should be done?

At the end of his research review, Sinclair suggests:

> In general the findings pose problems rather than suggest solutions. Research has shown that the main policies on residential care for the elderly have not worked out as intended. It has not shown how the policies can be made to work, or what policies would be 'better'.

... In considering the size and clientele of the residential sector, the committee may note the evidence that additional residential places are likely to be filled but many of those who fill them will probably not want or in a sense 'need' to be there. Conversely a reduction in the number of places might be a rash step given the evidence of unmet demand and the predicted increase in 'need'. One possible policy would therefore seek a 'standstill' in the number of residential places for the elderly (a difficult policy to implement given the problems of controlling the growth of the private residential sector without reducing the sector itself), and a determined effort to ensure that old people do not enter the homes if they would prefer not to and alternative arrangements can be made for them. Given the determined implementation of such a policy, a more accurate assessment of need for places might be made.

... Much of the evidence suggests (to me) the need for sheltered housing complexes with additional facilities (i.e. more staff, close liaison with domiciliary nursing staff, short-term assessment flats with vacancies for emergencies, a day centre and perhaps a small residential unit for the 'confused', many of whom seem to try the patience of all providers of care).

Such condensed comment reveals the complexity of the policy issues which are involved in decisions about the future of residential care. These include:

1. the improvement of community care services to elderly people and their carers in their own homes;
2. more effective cooperation between housing, the social service departments and the health service;
3. a strategy concerning the part to be played by private care in meeting need and the extent to which that market should be regulated.

There are other less tangible factors; for example, the extent to which old people feel safe in the area in which they live affects demand (meals-on-wheels do not make up for burglars!). Furthermore, development of local authority sheltered housing is bound up with wider issues of housing policy and with the role of private or voluntary housing schemes.

Thus the ripples spread wider and wider into fields of social policy, critically affected by political ideology and resource constraints. Even if the desired directions were agreed, it would take until the end of the century, and beyond, significantly to change the physical structure of provision, towards sheltered housing and associated services of the kind which Sinclair suggested. Meanwhile, old people need help now. What is urgently needed is a firm and consistent lead from central government, based on a political consensus of the kind which led in the 1970s to agreement on pension schemes, (but on which the present government, sadly, reneged). As with pension schemes, policies involving capital expenditure on housing provision of whatever kind, require long-range planning, as does the balance between different types of care and support. It cannot be subjected to 'stop-go' political manœuvres.

One nettle which will have to be grasped concerns the place of private residential care in overall provision. This is likely to be one of the most contentious issues politically. The growth of private care in the past decade has been spectacular as Table 7.1 has shown.

It is important to distinguish between the debate about the volume of private care and about its quality. So far as volume is concerned, there seem to be three problems. Firstly, as mentioned earlier and as the Audit Commission (1986) forcefully pointed out, large sums of public money have gone to supporting old people in such homes, which might otherwise have been used for community care – the preferred way of life for most. About half the residents in private homes are thus supported. This matter has been explored by the Firth Committee (DHSS, 1987) whose recommendations are currently under consideration. There is ample evidence that many old people do not choose private care in any meaningful way, nor are they even consulted – the arrangements being made by professionals or relatives (Weaver *et al.*, 1985). Therefore, it is arguable that unchecked growth in private care distorts public policy and denies old people legitimate alternatives.

Secondly, the location of private care has been more determined by available housing than by the needs of old people in a particular area. This has unfortunate consequences; it may lead old people to leave familiar areas and to distance themselves from relatives and friends who, as they grow old, find it increasingly difficult to visit. Rapid growth in some areas, such as seaside towns, with boarding houses suitable for conversion, distorts provision and creates quite abnormal concentrations of old people.

Thirdly, the sheer size of the increase has posed serious problems for the registering authorities and thereby threatened quality control, to which we now turn.

Discussions about quality tend to polarise, with comments (and horror stories) about the deficiencies of public sector provision set against those about the private sector. This is unhelpful and often reflects an ideological predisposition to see good in one sector rather than another.

There are intractable problems in providing through residential care in either sector an environment which is secure, stimulating and flexible, and which allows old people the degree of autonomy of which they are capable. The framework of statutory provision, within the local authority, poses the particular problems associated with bureaucratic control. The private sector is not thus constrained. However, other constraints operate in that sector. Most of the evidence currently available concerns rest homes rather than nursing homes, but with both, of course, this matter of profit margins looms large. Most of the rest homes which have opened in the 1980s are relatively small and their owners, therefore, need to keep their numbers up to the maximum wherever possible. Furthermore, since staff costs are the major factor in breaking even, there is a constant temptation in small homes to cut these below an acceptable level, or for staff to work excessive hours. In many of the new rest homes the proprietor works as staff and, as Weaver *et al.* (1985) have shown, there is a danger of exhaustion and 'burn out' in these situations.

A second problem in private care concerns the premises. While the design of many local authority homes is rather dispiriting and unimaginative, many private homes are sound, comfortable buildings, formerly boarding or guest houses, which fit unobstrusively into the area. The problem is, however, that without considerable alterations, their internal design may be unsatisfactory for the accomodation of elderly residents and this can require substantial expenditure. In addition to expensive fire precautions, installation of the modifications to toilets and bathrooms and corridors to accomodate wheelchairs and walking aids, the construction of ramps, and so on, are sometimes problematic as well as expensive. Unfortunately, a number of those who have set up such homes have had insufficient understanding beforehand of what was involved.

Behind these practicalities lies a question which society must address as a matter of urgency. Is it right that anyone, regardless of qualification or experience, can buy and run a rest home for old people without any requirement to employ qualified staff? Can this be allowed to continue? Sinclair (1987) describes private homes in this country as 'part of a cottage industry'. Up to 70 per cent are run by husband and wife teams living on the premises, few of whom have relevant qualifications (whereas those in charge of local authority homes now are nearly all trained). Surely minimum educational and/or vocational qualifications should be laid down?

Local authority social service departments now have duties under the Registered Homes Act 1984 for the registration and inspection of such homes and they have, as guidance, the document *Home Life* (1985) which was drawn up by Lady Avebury's working party at the request of the then government. (Health Authorities have similar duties for nursing homes.) It is generally accepted that the principles in it are admirable, but that the present reality, in all sectors, falls far short of that ideal. Social service departments have the delicate (and sometimes embarrassing) task of comparing their provision to that of the private sector, for example in the number of rooms with two or more occupants as against the recommended single rooms. There is research evidence (Sinclair, 1987) that local authorities 'vary widely in commitment to the task of regulation'. The resource implications of doing this work well are considerable, especially for those authorities (health and local), many on the south coast, which have seen a sudden very large increase in registered homes. However, the problem is not merely one of resources. The extent to which authorities involve themselves in issues surrounding private care is also related to the local political climate and, more generally, to the level of interest and expertise in services to old people generally.

Be that as it may, these variations mean that old people and their relatives cannot know what to expect from a particular social service department, what registration really means in terms of quality control, beyond basic minimum requirements. Social workers are often instructed not to recommend rest or nursing homes, merely to supply a list of registered homes. That is a situation about which many, especially those who work in hospitals, feel very uncomfortable. It illustrates a kind of bureaucratic hypocrisy – on what basis has registration been granted if a home cannot be recommended? For these reasons, it has been suggested that there should be other methods of controlling quality, one of the most important of which potentially concerns the involvement of staff in the private sector in local authority training programmes.

If a local authority refuses to register, or withdraws registration from a home, the proprietors may appeal to the Registered Homes Tribunal, set up in 1984. There has been a rapid increase in such appeals but in a substantial majority of cases, the authority's decisions have been upheld. (The hearings are in public and the cases published.) Undoubtedly, there are some alarming examples of poor care. But that is not an argument against the very existence of private care – it draws attention to the dangers in rapid, uncontrolled expansion and to some of the particular difficulties which confront 'cottage industries'. There are indications that we shall soon see a trend from the USA towards 'groups' or 'chains' of rest homes and nursing homes, where some of the problems outlined above will not arise. However, no doubt there will be others, notably those connected with accountability between those who own and those who manage.

Little reference has been made in the foregoing discussion to the place of the voluntary sector in the provision of residential care. It is much smaller than public or private sectors and, as seen in Table 7.1, numbers have decreased slightly in the past decade, from 9.5 to 8.5 per thousand of the over 75s. In 1984, about 27 000 people were thus accommodated. However, it is known that the average age on admission to voluntary homes is rather lower so the total numbers are greater. Current preoccupation with the growth in private care has dampened discussion of voluntary homes. However, it is interesting to recall that Townsend (1964) found that although, at that time, the physical provision of many voluntary homes fell below that of the local authority, there was a higher degree of satisfaction amongst residents. This is no doubt attributable to the fact that a substantial proportion of these residents choose a home with which they have religious or professional affiliation or some other positive reason to do with a sense of belonging. Their importance, therefore, in the overall pattern of provision should not be underestimated. They may have an increasingly significant part to play in caring for ethnic minority groups of elderly people, as they have already done for elderly Jews, for example. This is an example of a legitimate extension of choice, by which groups of old people can live in an environment with familiar values, traditions and habits, all of which contribute to their security and fulfilment. Some contemporary detailed studies of such homes is overdue – if successful they may thrown much light on the factors necessary to create an acceptable residential environment.

There are then six assumptions which should underpin policy development in residential care.

1. There can be no dispute that progress on community care is urgently needed, if old people (most of whom want to stay at home) are to have real choice.
2. Where staying at home is not possible, flexible variations on the theme of sheltered housing, with additional readily available resources for various kinds of support, are likely to be the preferred alternative for many.
3. It is imperative that, centrally and locally, there should be strategic planning of the overall provision and distribution of residential care in all sectors.
4. The present financial anomalies between sectors must be sorted out.
5. Particular attention needs to be paid to residential provision for the severely mentally infirm, for whom this may be the only effective way of providing care and relieving carers.
6. Existing residential provision needs radical review, initiated by central government, for reasons to which we now turn.

Reference has already been made to the long standing problems which are widely recognised in providing care in institutional settings for vulnerable and dependent people. Of paramount importance is the danger of what may be termed 'institutional maintenance' becoming more important than the needs of residents. At their most excessive, procedures and routines are entirely geared to the needs of staff, the smooth-running of the institution and (in more or less explicit ways) to the control of the residents to prevent disruption or inconvenience to staff. Experience over many years, however, has shown that these tendencies exist even in forms of care which are overtly geared to providing a sensitive, home-like atmosphere for residents. Nor are they avoided simply by reduction in size. The Select Committee of the House of Commons (1985) notes this in respect of hostels for the mentally handicapped.

> Smallness of itself is no guarantee of a high quality of care: small is not necessarily beautiful. As Dr Simon of the NDTMHP observed 'Every unit has the danger of giving into institutionalisation, however gradually they do it. I have seen six-bedded houses thoroughly institutionalised, much more so than 24-bedded units.'

Similarly, it is a matter of common experience that some homes for old people seem dominated by such institutional procedures and routines. Complex processes are at work in producing this situation. Occupational background and training of staff has a bearing on their attitudes both to residents and to organisational matters. There is some evidence (King *et al.*, 1971) that hospital trained staff may tend to be inflexible in the way they construct regimes of care and that this behaviour may be carried into other residential settings, such as hostels or homes. The extent to which certain routines and systems are necessary within hospitals cannot be fully explored here. Clearly, in high risk, life and death situations, such as are found in acute medical or surgical wards, and for the protection of patients against unnecessary risk (for example, in the administration of drugs), firm and established patterns of work are essential. Even so, the anxiety engendered by the work can lead to an excessive preoccupation with checks and routines (Menzies, 1970).

Many staff with hospital experience and training are now employed in care establishments and bring much that is of value to the work. However, in this particular respect, some of their occupational 'luggage' may be less helpful. Furthermore, they frequently have had little or no retraining for their new roles. It is easy to see how there may on occasions be an inappropriate transfer of hospital custom and practice to the world outside and how difficult it may be to modify an 'acute' hospital environment to the needs of long-stay residents.

It must be emphasised that anxiety about organisational accountability is not confined to care in hospitals. Local authority care operates within the normal constraints of a local government bureaucracy; for example, there have to be financial controls. Yet these can lead to practices which have the effect of demeaning residents, such as placing limits on the freedom of children or adolescents to buy clothes where they like or in the way old people's personal allowances are given to them.

In addition to matters concerning financial accountability, there is also legitimate concern about the protection of residents or patients. Thus certain fire precautions are required in residential establishments and not in domestic households. On occasion, they inconvenience residents, as when heavy fire doors impede the progress of the infirm. Obviously they are designed to protect against a terrible hazard. Yet in their own homes old people may smoke in their bedrooms; very few have so much as a fire extinguisher, let alone means of escape from upstairs rooms.

The keeping of records of fire drills is a logical consequence of the requirements, yet may be experienced by staff as another strain in the burden of paperwork which threatens to overwhelm and divert them from personal care of residents. Another example concerns the administration of drugs. Staff must have careful procedures for this and must keep records about it. Again, the reasons are obvious and seem amply justified. Yet hundreds of thousands of old people at home, a substantial number of whom are mentally frail, have very little help with taking the right pills at the right time. It is not likely at present that a local or health authority will be criticised if an old person dies, is injured or ill in his or her own home as a result of a fire or a drug accident. (Whether such criticism will be heard once community care plans for individuals are more widely made and understood will be interesting to see.) Yet society does appear to expect the state to protect people (of all kinds) against fire, who gather together in certain recognised ways and places, whether in schools, hospitals, football stadiums or old people's homes. Furthermore, it expects additional protection for those gathered together who are deemed incompetent or less competent, in certain matters such as control over medication.

All this is quite widely understood, yet the whole question of acceptable and unacceptable risks in residential care for old people is fraught with difficulty. (This has been excellently discussed by Norman (1980).) It undoubtedly has a significant bearing on the question of institutional maintenance. On the one hand it can rightly be argued that a good many of the precautions against risk are for the protection of residents, not staff. On the other hand, because staff feel accountable for accidents, there is a powerful tendency to seek to mini-mise risk to the point when resident's quality of life is jeopardized. This is when the fundamental objectives of the establishment get blurred. Thus, if a decision is taken that all medicine must be held centrally and not in residents' rooms, this may deprive a lucid and independent resident from exercising control over that domain of his or her life.

Achieving a proper balance between sensible safety and legitimate risk-taking is a challenge to staff at different levels in an establishment. Inevitably, however, it is staff in charge who bear the heaviest responsibility for finding that balance. To do so they need the support of management staff outside the home or the ward; in particular they need to be confident that they will be supported against criticism if accidents occur as a result of considered risks in a flexible regime. In that way, the anxieties will be held in check which can so easily lead to excessive preoccupation with protection of residents, and thence to practices which, through institutional rigidity, diminish the opportunity for residents to exercise choice.

Concern about external accountability is not, however, simply focused upon risks of accidents or misadventures. Standards of cleanliness and hygiene are also involved and may preoccupy staff to the point, as Willcocks *et al.* (1987) suggest, that they become the dominant goal. However, it is important not to underestimate their importance to the well-being of residents and for the image of the home. Furthermore, a group of old people which con-tains a number who are incontinent, presents a formidable task if they are to be comfortable and the institution sweet-smelling. Again, we see how, up to point, these activities are for the benefit of residents but, beyond that point, they work against it.

So far we have focused on the way previous experience of some staff, linked to feelings of public accountability for the care given, creates a concern for and anxiety about, safety and hygiene which may on occasion set in motion institutional practices which are inimical to the well-being of residents.

However, that is not the end of the story. Goffman's (1961) analysis of 'total institutions' (in that case, large mental hospitals) includes description of pro-cesses by which inmates were 'stripped' of their identity (such as taking away clothes on admission), and subjected to 'batch' living (in which their daily activities were regimented and timed). Some of the routines were so extreme as to seem bizarre. Yet when one examines the daily routines of residential institutions for old people, it is clear that there is the potential for similarly depersonalising procedures and that these are not simply attributable to matters concerning safety and risk taking. Why then do they occur?

The inescapable and depressing fact is that these processes derive from attitudes of carers to those being cared for. There are three elements in these: the tendency to stereotype; attribution of incompetence; and (explicitly or implicitly) an exploitation of unequal power.

The first two of these are bound up with attitudes to old people and reflect the 'ageism' which has been earlier discussed. Although stereotyping is not by definition dysfunctional, the process usually demeans because it is the negative aspects of the group in question which are stressed. In the case of old people, it may involve the attribution of characteristics to old people as a whole which denies them the right to be viewed and treated as individuals with distinctive and widely varying strengths, weaknesses and needs. The use of the word 'they' is revealing: 'they like to be/to do' and so on. Even when the content is positive, comments such as 'I like old people' have an empty, stereotypical quality. The attribution of incompetence is associated with stereotyping. It involves blanket assumptions concerning old people's incapacity to manage their affairs which are not based upon individual assessment.

As was discussed in the first chapter, one of the central problems in helping residential staff to avoid these dangers is that there are no clear norms of development in the last years of life as there are for children. The variations in physical and mental capacity between old people all aged 80 are often considerable, even in a residential group. Thus 'ageism' in residential care creates a climate in which depersonalising processes, embodied in procedure and routines, become easier to implement. Once old people are not viewed as individual adults the scene is set for insensitive practices. Much of the tension surrounding incontinence is linked to this. Bowel and bladder control are for us all symbols of adult status. As independent adults, we control these functions without much thought or anxiety – free 'to go' when we want. Physical frailty makes us dependent on others. If, in an institution, toilet arrangements are governed more by staff convenience than the widely varying needs of the residents, anxiety mounts to a distressing degree and has a ripple effect on morale in the home. Obviously, staff shortages play a part in creating these conditions, since they reduce the opportunity for individual interactions between staff and residents. Whilst adequate staffing levels are of critical importance in providing the conditions necessary for good practice, they are not sufficient in themselves. For that, fundamental attitudes have to be sound.

One should not underestimate the difficulties for staff in establishing and maintaining attitudes to the old people in their care which emphasise their individuality and build upon their competence in daily living. Almost by definition, the population in such homes is frail, with a substantial degree of physical and mental infirmity. Recent research, however, from a variety of sources including Booth (1985), suggests that, although there are a core of old people who are as dependent as those in hospital or nursing homes, there has been a tendency to exaggerate their actual numbers in proportion to the totality of residents. Certainly the 'received wisdom' of staff is that they are now looking after a greater and very high proportion of the severely dependent. If the research findings are upheld, it may indicate, as Booth suggests, that some residents are so demanding of time and energy that they 'loom too large'. However, this is also made more likely in an environment in which staff are failing adequately to distinguish between their residents' capacities.

It is particularly difficult for staff to individualise those residents with a degree of confusion, who lie in the middle of the continuum between total mental competence, and near-total incompetence. These are the people who have good and bad days, and who function better in some areas of daily living than in others. To adjust responses to their needs is a delicate matter.

So, the dominance of institutional maintenance over other goals is made more likely when old people (or, indeed, any other similar groups) are subject to stereotyping and assumptions of incompetence. What part does the imbalance of power play in this? The history of institutional care reveals all too starkly how unequal power can be exploited, sometimes in severe and frightening ways. It is not often that its sinister aspect is manifest in the care of old people. Yet even when a regime is essentially benign, the vulnerability of the residents, the fact that they often cannot fight back (physically or verbally), or even leave the room if annoyed, and that they have nowhere else to go, induces a degree of conformity which in turn encourages the dominance of institutional maintenance mechanisms. The very many committed and concerned staff in our homes would do well to place themselves imaginatively in residents' shoes. It is one of the paradoxes of residential care, that the various parties involved may all feel themselves to an extent powerless. Care staff, for example, may feel powerless to change practices dictated by those in charge. In other forms of institutional care, there may be fear of the residents who are known to be powerful in various ways. Adolescents and prisoners, for example, may get out of control. However, old people in homes have little power, real or perceived, in comparison. This is partly due to the physical and mental frailty which many endure, but there are other equally significant factors. Many old people, by virtue of their generation and social class, do not expect to 'call the tune', whether or not they 'pay the piper'. They expect to be grateful. The fact that so many are women increases a tendency to submissiveness outside their own domestic domain. Also, such woman are unlikely to be used to the exercise of group power, such as that of unions. It is rare for a group of residents to complain to management. Ironically, this is more likely when empowerment processes have been set in train by staff, through residents' committees and so on. Where they exist and flourish, they will inevitably challenge institutional maintenance ('why do we have to . . .?').

In the foregoing discussion, it was not the intention to deny or to disparage the strenuous efforts made by many residential staff to create an environment in which the needs of individual residents can be respected. However, it has to be acknowledged that there are powerful forces working against such initiatives and that much of the resistance can be attributed to the opposing drive towards institutional maintenance.

While some of the issues which must be confronted are general to all residential care, others are particular to old people's homes. One in particular has been emphasised by Willcocks *et al.* (1987) and concerns 'the physical world' of the home. Willcocks points out that most architectural briefs for such homes 'demand a compromise between domestic and institutional architecture. Yet many of the purpose built homes . . . (suggest) that architects have failed to reach such a reconciliation.'

> In contrast with the domestic home, these buildings fail to convey any sense of personal ownership, of territoriality, or of individual influence over external appearance. These are all features which suggest that the occupants are distanced from their environments. To the community at large, residential homes reinforce a view which conveys an impression that residents are a homogeneous group of 'old people' lacking personal identity or individuality.

Willcocks *et al.* further comment on the internal spatial arrangements in their research study of local authority homes. They found that only half the residents had single bedrooms and many had to use public spaces to see their visitors. They discuss the well-known phenomenon of 'chairs round the walls' of the lounge and comment that:

> There is, after all, no reason why residents – generally strangers to each other – should wish to engage in continuous interaction, especially when they may be sitting in the same seats for up to eight hours a day. If this period were not so long then interaction might be more acceptable. The 'backs to the wall' strategy may be construed as a retreat position, and the somewhat uninterested focusing upon the television as a further strategy for avoiding eye contact with other residents.

Control of the immediate environment was also important to residents. Yet in matters deemed by residents to be important, opening windows and doors, storage space, good sound insulation between rooms, and a power point in the bedroom, 'the scope for personal control was very basic and available to only a minority of residents'. Similar points are made about negotiability, being able to get round the home easily. Willcocks *et al.* conclude:

> It is of major concern that the 1970s purpose-built homes are characterized by obstacles to mobility which are traditionally associated with older homes. Although problems associated with access to bedrooms, bathrooms, and toilets show a marked diminution in new homes, crucial

areas of mobility such as manœuvrability through doorways and along corridors continue to create difficulties for physically frail residents.

Apart from the considerable value in having the detail of these matters so well documented, this research is invaluable in drawing attention to aspects of the residents' environment which are not under the direct control of staff, yet crucially affect the degree of autonomy which frail people can exercise.

Whilst some of the design flaws arise from resource constraints and yet others from preoccupation with perceived staff needs, some arise from a lack of imagination and from a failure to apply what we know for ourselves in everyday life to old people's desires and needs. Thus, restaurants and open plan offices frequently provide personal space by judicious use of dividers, plants and so on. Storage space is highly prized by those who buy houses. The matters felt to be important by the old people in Willcocks' survey are important to all of us, with two significant extra dimensions. Old people stay indoors much more and their living space is even more important. They are more often dependent on aids to walking or on wheelchairs and access is therefore critical.

Thus we can see that quality of life in residential care is not only dependent on staff attitudes, vital as these are. It is also inextricably tied to the details of the physical environment. However, while agreeable conditions enhance quality of life, most old people would probably rate their daily contact with staff as of even more importance. Staff have the power to make life pleasant, tolerable, miserable or intolerable. Sadly, the picture that emerges from Willcocks' research is a depressing one. The researchers comment on the centrality of domestic and cleaning activities in the lives of care and domestic staff and find that social care assumes a secondary position.

> For neither day or night care staff was there any question of putting aside domestic chores in order to enter into social exchange with residents.

It has been earlier suggested it is important to acknowledge the importance of cleanliness for residents' psychological well-being. Yet it seems clear from Willcocks' research that the balance between these elements in care is wrong. The ordinary human need for social interactions with staff is increased by the fact that old people in homes often have little contact with anyone else and because the quality of their interaction with other residents is patchy.

Many factors are at work in this, including the question of accountability, earlier discussed. Cleaning and domestic activity has high visibility whereas social interaction does not. Staff feel themselves under pressure to keep up with physical care tasks; given time constraints, it is these which are accorded priority. Yet there are other less obvious problems. It is not easy to interact constructively with old people, with varying degrees of mental competence and difficulties in communication, such as deafness. More fundamental still, ageist assumptions diminish meaningful exchanges. Banal, patronising and mechanical responses all too easily prevail in the interactions.

It must be emphasised that the attitudes of many care staff are no different from those in the general population. Indeed they mirror them. Kindness and warmth are often demonstrated so far as the structure of the work permits or encourages. It is particularly difficult to relate meaningfully, if the residents have no known past. Conversely, where the old people and care assistants come from a stable community, the two groups may have knowledge of each other which facilitates communication. Many care staff have not been offered, through training, the opportunity to learn how to make good social contact with unfamiliar old people. Until very recently care staff have been paid as unskilled manual workers, a grading which reflects the low status of the work. As discussed in Chapter 4, this in turn is bound up with social ambivalence about work which has a 'tending' component involving physical care. This is both idealised, as in 'motherhood', and devalued, as, for example, in nurses' pay. Such work is, of course, usually carried out by women.

We are a very long way from creating a social climate in which the value of tending work is recognised and the resources unlocked to recompense and train adequately those who perform it. Perhaps controversially, it is suggested here that the deficiencies in local authority provision do not mainly lie in a shortage of staff but in the way which they are deployed and the lack of appreciation of the skills required to do a job in which physical and social care are sensitively combined.

It is generally accepted, of course, that senior staff in charge have a critical role in creating the regime of the home; without their assent or encouragement, external influences are of no avail. Willcocks *et al.* (1987) found that 42 per cent had no relevant qualification, although as mentioned earlier, most officers in charge now hold a relevant qualification. The most likely vocational qualification was in nursing (the difficulties of which were earlier discussed); only a handful had a social work qualification. The authors suggest that the role of such staff was characterised by preoccupation with administrative tasks rather than with the creation of the residential climate. Such administrative work derives from local authority requirements and is as important in terms of public accountability as hygiene or cleanliness. Administrative competence is highly desirable. It can help to create conditions which are stable, which help old people to feel safe and which actually help to individualise residents, for example, through the keeping of good records about them. Yet it can be 'a retreat into the office' and so easily becomes a dominant feature of institutional maintenance.

In writing this account of the difficulties and dilemmas which beset residential care, I have been keenly aware of those in such work who may read this book and who may feel discouraged or angry at the negative impression it conveys. Paradoxically, it is likely to be those most concerned to learn and to improve care for residents who read such books. Residential staff in general have become accustomed to criticism and to doubts about their very *raison d'être*. That there is confusion and ambivalence is illustrated by the fact that the government has set up a committee (chaired by Lady Wagner and hosted by the National Institute of Social Work) to examine the position, and which has recently reported (NISW, 1988). So far as residential care of old people is concerned, it is hard to avoid the conclusion reached by Willcocks *et al.* that radical restructuring rather than remedial action is called for. The evidence from a wide body of research is compelling and seems to point that way. They summarise the broad thrust of this radical reform for local authority homes as follows:

1. Innovation or adaptation of the physical form of homes to establish access to and control over personal territory for elderly people.
2. Changes in social arrangements and management within homes to define individual rights and acceptable risks; homes must respond in practical terms to the demands of 'normalization'.
3. An alternative management structure for social services departments to integrate service provision and service delivery for old people in the community and in the residential section – this must expose the arbitrary nature of the institutional boundary.
4. Revised training schemes for field and residential staff, both management and workers, to support this alternative form of institutional care as one option within the community care spectrum.
5. Changes in community influence on the running of homes and involvement in activities within the homes; this must be a major part of democratizing services and encouraging communities to win back the welfare institutions that historically they have subscribed to but never owned.

Can residential staff and those who manage them see such proposals as a challenge, an opportunity for action to the end of the century and beyond, rather than reacting defensively to the criticism of the status quo?

The third and fifth of the proposals offer opportunities which are to some extent being grasped. In other fields, in particular in child care, the boundaries between residential and community provision have been deliberately blurred, as in the development of family centres. There is now increasing discussion of the use of old people's homes as resource centres. The potential activities and outreach of such centres is diagrammatically illustrated in Fig. 7.1.

Such a concept might revolutionalise the place of a home in the local community; even when they are sited on estates, the isolation of so many homes at present is patent. It would be particularly valuable for informal carers to find in the home a ready source of support and advice. However, such a model could easily neglect the needs of permanent residents. Innovations and exciting schemes could proliferate and the residents be left stranded on a lonely island while busy project workers sailed in and out of the harbour. There can be no substitute for systematic and detailed consideration of their social and emotional needs and the environment which will best meet them. Furthermore, if it is to be their home, residents need space which is private and safe

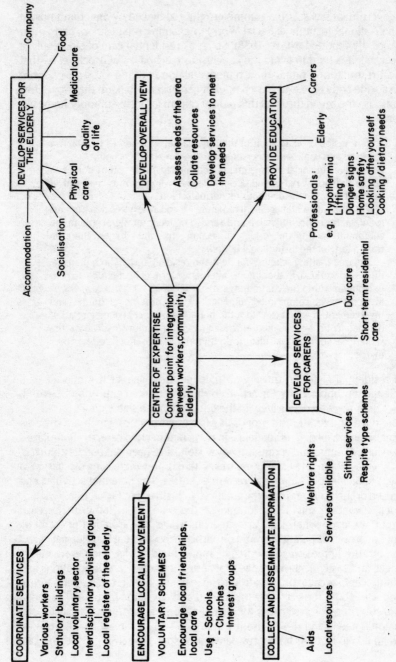

Fig. 7.1 Role of a centre of expertise. (By permission of J. Bromley. Internal Document for Doncaster Social Services Department, 1986.)

from invasion by outsiders (however stimulating), and from excessive bustle and noise. This has quite complex implications for the use or extension of existing establishments.

In conclusion, the history of residential care for elderly people, as others, is a chequered one. It has proved extremely difficult to provide an environment which upholds the dignity of old people and to find an appropriate balance between risk and security. There is evidence from both the statutory and private sectors that all is not well and the rapid growth of the latter has created serious difficulties in quality control. Although the evidence suggests that most old people would prefer to have their own front door, in one way or another, rather than live in residential care, the policy and resource implications are so great that we will continue to need residential care for the foreseeable future. Therefore, it is urged that attention be given to the radical reforms advocated by Willcocks *et al.* Above all, the quality and training of staff should be recognised as of paramount importance. The resources necessary to raise staffing standards must be unlocked. Old people in residential care are amongst the most vulnerable and dependent in society. Our claim to be a compassionate society should be judged by the efforts we make to ensure their peace and comfort at the end of their lives.

CHAPTER 8

Issues for the next decade

As will be apparent from the earlier chapters, the issues for the future are many and complex, as are their interactions. It would be tedious simply to reiterate them in this concluding chapter. Those on which I have chosen to comment are inevitably subjective and their choice somewhat arbitrary but must surely be regarded as amongst the most important.

This chapter considers firstly the specific issues arising from four care areas of provision – income maintenance, housing and health; secondly, organisational and structural problems in community care; thirdly, the role of social service departments; fourthly, the position of ethnic minorities; lastly, the problem of mental illness in old age.

The link between all these issues is a profound concern about the status of very old people in our society at the end of the twentieth century. As we have seen, ageism is endemic; it is 'institutionalised', as is racism. Many whose attitudes are, at a personal level, quite benign, do not challenge assumptions about the inferior positions of old people in society and about their capabilities. It is critical that practitioners working with old people show increased awareness, and raise it in others, of the process by which old people are demeaned, stigmatised and deprived of choice.

Income maintenance, housing and health are central to the well-being of frail old people. All three are increasingly problematic.

Income maintenance

In Chapter 2, we discussed the notion of structured dependency and showed how this is bound up with poverty. The next 15 years will see the effects of the social security reforms, in particular the changes in the State Earnings Related Pension Scheme and projected growth in private and occupational pension schemes. Unless the current government changes course, we shall see the continuance of a flat rate pension linked to the rise in prices, not earnings, which increases the gap between the better off and the poor. For a substantial minority of the very poor, we shall see the new income support scheme replacing supplementary benefit and the workings of the new discretionary Social Fund replacing single payments. As the years go by, there will be a new generation of pensioners whose earnings were interrupted or prematurely ended through unemployment and who have not therefore acquired the material comforts and security for which they had hoped and worked.

Political attitudes towards income maintenance and old people are ambivalent and sometimes hypocritical. They are a substantial part of the electorate and they attract public sympathy, so they cannot be ignored. Yet relatively small increases in social security provision have significant implications for public expenditure and governments of any colour are likely to be cautious about improving the lot of pensioners.

Whilst political change may alter the emphasis of policy, it is hard to avoid the conclusion that for the foreseeable future, a very large section of the elderly population will not share in the nation's increasing wealth, that they will remain an under-class, conditioned by repeated references to them as burdens, to ask for little and to be grateful. Their structured dependency is assured.

This depressing prediction implies that the practitioners, of whatever discipline, will often be called upon to 'limit the damage', to find ways of improving people's income, through welfare rights activity, for example, or to find alternative means of improving their lot, which do not demean the recipient.

Housing

Arguably, it is in the sphere of housing that most can and must be done. 'Housing poverty' amongst old people is a social disgrace and is probably responsible for more anxiety and unhappiness than lack of money in the pocket. Taylor (1986) has analysed the position of elderly owner occupiers, a matter much neglected until recently. He points out that just over half of elderly households are in some form of owner occupation and that this proportion can be expected to rise, possibly to 70 per cent, by the end of the century.

> A number of studies in recent years have revealed that there are large numbers of very elderly people living alone in houses which are difficult to maintain and often unsuited to their daily needs. Nearly a quarter (24 per cent) of all households in Great Britain comprise only elderly people of whom around one-third live alone. As a consequence of the differences in lifespan, two-fifths of elderly home-owners are women who live alone,

and 35 per cent of them are aged over 75. Although a slight fall is expected in the 'younger' retired group over the next 30 years, this imbalance is likely to increase, since the number of those aged 75 or over is estimated to rise still further, while the number of those who have reached 85 years or over is likely to double. There are also many retired couples who, although physically fit, nevertheless live in accommodation which is too large for them. They too have begun to calculate the long-term benefits of moving into smaller, more convenient property. Until recently there has been only fitful recognition of changes taking place in respect of house-hold composition in this country, so that the needs of the rapidly expand-ing group of elderly owner-occupiers have not, for the most part, been catered for.

Taylor discusses the voluntary, private and statutory initiatives which have begun to emerge as a response to the problem. There are two broad options. One is to move to smaller, convenient, sometimes sheltered housing.

Another consists of assistance with improvements and repairs to elderly people's existing homes in order to enable them to 'stay-put' comfortably. These and other approaches suggest that the outline of a comprehensive policy for meeting the needs of elderly home-owners already exists; what is needed is an injection of funding and central direction to co-ordinate the effort.

Taylor recommends the establishment of a housing agency service within local authorities, supported by central government.

A complete housing agency service would comprise four elements: knowledge both of the needs of the local elderly population and the resources available to meet them; publicity and information about what is available and where to go in order to get it; advice and help in respect of individual problems, and long term support in those cases that require it.

It remains to be seen whether such a proposal finds political favour, locally or centrally. What Taylor demonstrates beyond doubt is that the confusion and fragmentation of responsibility at present is quite unacceptable and places at risk many elderly people who are perplexed and worried about their homes, which they have striven to buy. The independence which they so prized as owner occupiers can paradoxically become a source of increased dependence on others when they cannot manage the house or the garden or negotiate the stairs. It is good to see that this aspect of social policy seems to be attracting increasing attention and that initiatives to give advice on 'staying-put' are being encouraged by central government, sparked off, perhaps, by Wheeler's (1982) pioneering research with the Anchor Trust.

Tinker (1984) studied new initiatives designed to help old people stay in their own homes. Her focus of attention was on alarm systems and on various forms of paid carers, who provided additional support to such people. Her important, detailed and carefully researched conclusions cannot here be repeated, but four merit particular emphasis. Firstly, the elderly people in the survey, one fifth of whom were either permanently bedfast or housebound, were more frail and older than those in sheltered housing. Secondly, despite that, nearly all of them wanted to stay in their own homes. Thirdly, they needed other forms of support to complement the innovatory schemes studied. Fourthly, some of these schemes were playing a crucial role in keeping people at home and were cost effective, though not cheap.

Fuel poverty

Closely associated with 'housing poverty' is 'fuel poverty'. Keeping warm enough is probably the single most worrying issue for a large proportion of old people. The emotive issue of hypothermia should not deflect us from facing the uncomfortable fact that very large numbers of old people live in unreasonably cold conditions which are well below recommended temperature. Research undertaken by Wicks (1978) is worth the attention of all those involved in direct care of old people in the community. (There is, unfortunately, a dearth of more recent evidence on the incidence of hypothermia and unacceptably cold conditions.) Wicks' findings have been explored by the author (Stevenson, 1988) in more detail but, in summary, his study revealed:

1. that the majority in a large survey had livingroom or bedroom temperatures below recommended levels;
2. nearly 10 per cent of the sample were at risk of developing hypothermia;
3. a complex and fascinating finding, 'poverty was not directly related to low care temperature but the receipt of Supplementary Benefit was'.

> Wicks showed that the room temperatures of those receiving supplementary benefit were not on average lower than those with higher incomes. But a significantly higher proportion of these claimants had dangerously low body temperatures. Of these, the very aged were the most vulnerable. Wicks concludes 'this is probably due to the effects of a declining physiology, perhaps exacerbated by illness, combined with the most deprived social conditions' (p.164). This finding cries out for further investigation, concerning the long-term effects of physical deprivation on the bodies of the aged and the impact of other contemporaneous factors such as clothing and nutrition.   (Stevenson, 1988)

Until such time as housing is routinely insulated and heated (as it is in Scandinavian countries) at a level safe and comfortable for old people, policies of community care fall at the first fence.

It is clear that housing policy, and its associated services designed to support frail people, interacts crucially with the provision of residential care in all sectors. An increasing residential sector may tell one as much about deficiencies in housing and support as it does about a demand for that form of provision. The present position is so unsatisfactory that it is creating a false market, for which, at present, both the state (through social security) and the individual (through the sale of their house) pay dearly. The restriction on local authority capital expenditure and its political overtones makes it improbable that much progress will be made in the area of statutory sheltered housing provision. There has, however, been a burgeoning of voluntary and private sheltered housing projects which can take their place amongst options for some elderly people. The fact remains, however, that a substantial majority will stay put, in homes which they own or rent. It is to their needs that urgent and sustained attention must now be given.

Health care

Turning to health, a curtain is raised on an array of problems, often intractable and bound up with the resourcing of the National Health Service and its competing priorities. These are beyond the remit of this book but, given its focus on the frail, it would be perverse not to reflect upon the importance of health issues in a concluding chapter. For practitioners, there would seem to be a number of key topics over which they have some measure of influence, according to their role, and it is on these we now reflect.

Firstly, one battle to be fought against ageism concerns assumptions about health in old age. Society generally still does not adequately distinguish between disease and frailty, between the remediable and the irremediable in old age. The failure to do so causes much unnecessary suffering. It is to be hoped that practitioners in health and social care will be in the forefront of social education programmes for the elderly and their carers.

Secondly, and closely allied, the potential of preventive health care is great and largely untapped. Leaving aside the importance of health education in earlier years for later well-being, there is also a more specific and focused job to be done with people in old age whose nutrition, failing eyesight or hearing (to take but three examples) may place them at unnecessary risk or discomfort. As mentioned earlier, the patchiness of age/sex registers in general practice is an unnecessary obstacle to sensible, modest screening programmes for the over 70s, whose health is at greater risk. The objections often raised to mass screening programmes for younger people do not apply, and there is ample evidence that health hazards are higher. It is difficult to believe earlier intervention would not be cost effective.

Thirdly, practitioners will often become involved in the interactions between hospital and community services. We have been very slow to follow through the implications of an ageing hospital population in terms of hospital discharge practices, accident and emergency provision and so on. Not all the problems are caused by bed shortage, some are sheer lack of imagination. Yet inappropriate speed in discharge and inadequate assessment of home circumstances can cause expensive readmission. The long-term effects of poorly managed admission and discharges may not have been widely evaluated but it is likely that they have detrimental effects on morale and confidence.

There is also growing awareness of the problems which can arise from over-use or misuse of drugs amongst elderly people. Such drugs can, of course, be prescribed or bought over the counter. (There is little evidence of illegal drug abuse amongst elderly people although it is suggested that alcoholism is on the increase.) Iatrogenic illness (that is, illness caused by medication) is well understood and much discussed but there are a number of factors which make it of particular concern amongst old people. One is that old people are prescribed more drugs than younger people and are much more likely to be taking four or more at the same time (apart from what they get from the chemist!) (Skegg *et al.*, 1986). Their interaction will on occasions be problematic. We know comparatively little of the effects of certain drugs in later life. There is little advice from drug companies about the dosage which may be appropriate for old people (as compared with children), yet some evidence that there are significant variations in the absorption and elimination of drugs in old age and their effects. A given dose in an elderly person may produce higher plasma or tissue concentrations over longer periods of time, thus causing, in effect, 'overdosing'. Accidental drug misuse is certain to be higher amongst very old people, especially those who live alone, a substantial proportion of whom will have a degree of mental confusion. Burns and Phillipson (1986) report that the use of sedatives and minor tranquillisers has risen by 66 per cent in the last 20 years, especially amongst elderly people.

Thus we have a growing problem with many serious and sometimes tragic consequences. The Royal College of Physicians (1984) has suggested that drug reactions are responsible, wholly or in part, for 10 per cent of the admissions to geriatric units. Accidents in the home, with long-term consequences for well-being, are not infrequently due to drug reactions; for example, sedative drugs can cause unsteadiness. Less well understood are the strange reactions to drugs which may on occasion produce bizarre behaviour, distressing to relatives, which is entirely atypical in the person concerned.

These brief comments open up an area of which all practitioners, medical and non-medical, should be acutely conscious. The responsibility for prescribing lies in the hands of the doctors and it is to be hoped that the profession, especially general practitioners, will become more aware of the need for increased vigilance on these matters. However, others who work with old people need to take this factor into account in making assessments and plans, and quite often may need to seek medical advice. It is all too easy for behaviour to be attributed to age or ill-health which is in fact 'drug induced'. Sadly, this discussion also reminds us that drugs may be used inappropriately to 'damp down' anxiety or sadness which is understandable in the context of the old person's social situation and which would be better alleviated by other means.

Structural problems

As was discussed in the chapter on formal community care, interprofessional cooperation is critical in service provision to old people. However, professionals do not work in an organisational vacuum and interagency collaboration provides the essential underpinning to individual activity. There are grounds for serious concern that our present arrangements are ineffective and inefficient.

The most significant of the structural interactions are between the health service, housing departments and social service departments. The complexity of the position is well illustrated in Fig. 8.1.

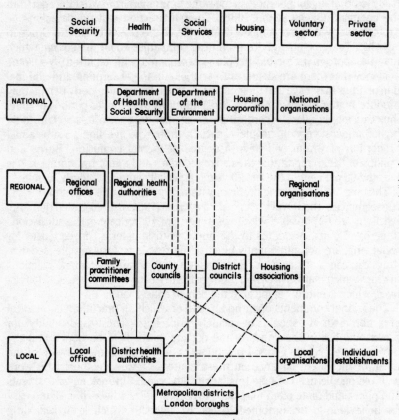

Fig. 8.1 Structural interactions between health service, housing departments and social service departments: —— indicates direct line responsibility, ---- indicates interrelationship. (Redrawn from Audit Commission, 1986).

The Audit Commission (1986) in their report *Making a Reality of Community Care* has sharply criticised the present structures and systems. They say that:

> The present management arrangements do not promote the essential integrated service and operational planning. In particular:
> (i) The structure of local community-based services is confused, with responsibility and accountability for elements of the services fragmented between different tiers of the NHS and within local government.
> (ii) As a result, the joint planning arrangements need to be complex and are particularly time-consuming to operate to ensure adequate liaison between all the various interests involved.
> (iii) The difficulties posed by the confused structure and complex planning arrangements are compounded by the lack of incentives and differences in the organisation styles of the different agencies concerned.
>
> Each of these problems might be soluble in isolation; but, together, they have combined to make it extraordinarily difficult to manage the transition to community-based care at the local level.

Although they acknowledge and analyse the interaction of the three components – national, regional and local, it is on the last of the three that we here concentrate since this is the 'sharp end' as far as practitioners are concerned and, as the Audit Commission recognises, 'the organisational arrangements for delivering care in the community reach their most complex at the local level'.

In a penetrating analysis, the Commission shows how the present formulation and organisational confusion works against effective provision. They point out that although many different agencies are involved, there is also 'day to day convergence between the services provided by the health service and local authority personal social service departments'. That is to say, there is lack of clarity about boundaries. For example, home help services may overlap with community nursing; district council housing departments are employing personnel as wardens and welfare officers whose roles may overlap with social services personnel. When boundaries are unclear, gaps and overlaps may lead to professional friction and to insecure old people.

As part of a strategy to overcome organisational separation, complex joint planning arrangements have evolved, of whose effectiveness the Audit Commission is pessimistic, seeing

> a number of difficulties inherent in placing responsibility for community care on such a mechanism. . . . If one of the agencies involved does not (or cannot) cooperate, at best any subsequent action will be delayed or distorted with key elements missing: at work, there will be no action at all. Such ragged or disjointed progress was one of the most common features observed.

They point out that the problems in joint planning are greatest where health, housing and social service boundaries do not coincide. Perhaps the most trenchant part of their critique, and one which suggests that radical change is needed, concerns the present lack of incentives for cooperation an an organisational level.

> Developing new services is hard work – especially if the main beneficiary is perceived to be some other agency. (Yet) . . . particularly at times of economic restraint and retrenchment, management are not penalised for failing to develop services. Rather they are congratulated for keeping costs down.

Thus we have a situation in which there are actually *disincentives* to cooperate at managerial level, yet the rhetoric of community care is all about initiatives and innovatory projects, many of which depend on the availability of finance from the different sectors. The Audit Commission's remedy is a contentious one, and rather unlikely to find political favour. They conclude that

> the objective of any changes should be to create an environment in which locally integrated community care can flourish. The present statutory framework constitutes a barrier.

Therefore:

> For care of elderly people in the community a single budget in an area should be established by contributions from the NHS and local authorities, the amount to be determined in each case by a formula agreed centrally. This budget should be under the control of a single manager who will purchase from whichever public or private agency he sees fit the appropriate services for elderly people in the community in the areas for which he is responsible. The manager's activities should be overseen by a small joint board of NHS and local authority representatives.

The merits of such a proposal and possible alternatives cannot here be argued. Indeed, Sir Roy Griffiths, in the recently published report on community care (1988), side-stepped the issue. What is important, however, is an appreciation of the organisational factors which make work at field level harder, which frustrate rather than facilitate the initiatives so urgently required.

Working within these frameworks are the practitioners. As the Commission points out,

> staff are the key resource for community care . . . sound manpower planning and effective training are thus essential. Unfortunately, both appear conspicuous by their absence as far as community care is concerned.

They point in particular to the dearth of occupational therapists who they see as central to the implementation of community care. However, they suggest that a manpower planning approach which is too rigidly tied to existing professional groups is unhelpful and 'a core of community care skills could be developed for all those involved in community based care based on shared training'.

However, it has to be said that all experience so far shows how intractable are the problems associated with interprofessional training at the basic qualifying level. It would seem that more progress is likely to be made by the development of post-qualifying and in-service training with an interprofessional/interagency focus, especially if this could be developed at local level with groups of practitioners who already have to work together and who may therefore see more readily the importance of such activities.

Such training programmes should have two separate but related elements. The first would be to increase understanding of frail elderly people in the community and of the support which they need. The previous chapters of this book direct attention to some of the most important matters. The second element would be to raise the awareness of those involved of the need for, and problems associated with, interagency and interprofessional work. This is a matter to which much attention is currently devoted in other areas of work such as child abuse. Numerous inquiries into the deaths of children have pointed to failures in such communication and cooperation which may have contributed to the tragedy.

Whilst one would not wish to expose practitioners who work with old people to the public scrutiny which has put child abuse workers under such stress, it seems likely that failures in cooperative activity leading to death or unnecessary emergencies would be uncovered if investigations took place. Less dramatic but of great importance, such failures may lead to distress and anxiety on the part of the old people and their carers. It is time that the importance of this aspect of professional activity is given the recognition which it deserves.

Role of social service departments

The third matter for consideration concerns the role of social service departments. The foregoing discussion has shown how much depends on them, both in terms of the direct provision of service and on their capacity to develop strategic planning across the sectors. Within our present structure they have a key role. Yet, as things stand at present, there are grounds for concern that they will not be able to play their role effectively. There are three main reasons for this. There can be little doubt that resource constraints seriously inhibit the development of community care initiatives. Whatever scope there is for more efficient use of existing resources, the need for additional expenditure on services for elderly people is clear, given demographic trends and no decrease in the needs of other client groups.

Social service departments have been subject to intensive internal competing pressures for available funds, notably in relation to child abuse but also to other community care groups, mentally ill and handicapped. Where hospital closure is imminent, a sense of urgency is created which continuing support for those at home does not engender. Although their numbers and the costs of residential and home help services keeps their share of the budget high, elderly people may lose out in the battle for increased resources for innovation and experiment.

Social workers outside hospitals have not had a particularly good record in work with elderly people; such work is frequently given to social work assistants. The creation of social service departments in 1970 has not resulted in generic social work service of any meaningful kind. For example, elderly clients are not assessed in the same way as children and families, with the same attention to their social and emotional situation (Chapter 6 on assessment is an attempt to set the record straight and offer guidance to practitioners about the values and assumptions which should underpin it.) There have been some hopeful developments, both on departments with local, 'patch' teams and those which have moved to specialist models. The lessons from these seems to be that 'generic' social workers with individual case loads cannot, almost by definition, maintain a balanced effort across all client groups. Some will be neglected, either because of worker preference of the departmental pressures or even political priorities. At present, there are signs of greatly increasing interest in old people amongst social work students, when such matters as are discussed in this book are put before them. In particular, feminists are challenged by the combination of ageism and sexism to which so many old women are subjected. However, unless service delivery is organised to give expression to such interest, it is bound to fade. Much depends on the attitude of managers. The problem is not simply one of sharing out scarce resources. Social workers need tangible signs that the quality of their work with old people is under review and that post-qualifying training is provided.

A concluding chapter on policy issues concerning social security, housing, health and the personal social services, which did not emphasise the need for increased resources, would be readily dismissed. Practitioners are keenly and painfully aware of resource constraints in their daily work. Party politics aside (and without entering the futile debates about the proper levels of increase in public expenditure), it is now widely accepted by all shades of informed opinion, recently powerfully confirmed by the Audit Commission, that public expenditure on services for elderly people is neither adequate nor properly directed at the present time. Whilst there will always be overriding constraints, influenced by the economic position and by the prevailing political ideology, those who read this book may share the author's view that there are fundamental questions of social morality now at stake. The respect we accord old people cannot be divorced from the money we are prepared to spend on them.

Old people in ethnic minorities

We turn now to two quite different matters to which reference has already been made, but which merit separate consideration. The first concerns the position of old people in ethnic minorities. Why should they be singled out? They are a very small proportion of the population of the very old in this country. We do not have reliable estimates of the numbers. In the 1981 census, persons of personable age from the New Commonwealth or Pakistan, accounted for less than 4 per cent of those households, compared with 17.4 per cent of all persons in England and Wales (DHSS, 1981). However, there are the other groups from European ethnic minorities, such as Poles, Ukranians and Jews, whose average age is higher, so that taken as a whole, the percentage will be rather higher. (For example, 18 per cent of Jews in this country are above retirement age.) Nevertheless, the numbers, proportionately and absolutely, are small.

The justification for special emphasis is fivefold.

1. The demographic trend can be predicted. We know that there will be a sharp increase in the numbers of the very old in such groups. Therefore, we have a rare opportunity to plan ahead. It will be a disgrace if we do not take that opportunity.
2. As Norman (1985) has pointed out, a number of such settlers, who are not yet of advanced age, suffer now from disabilities and disadvantages commonly associated with ageing.
3. As earlier discussed (Chapter 5), these elderly people are in 'triple jeopardy'.
4. Although nationally numbers are small, the concentration of some groups in certain parts of the country creates a distinctive and locally widespread need for particular provision. (For example, there are about 35 000 Cypriots (Turkish and Greek) living in the London Borough of Haringey, out of a total borough population of 228 000. A substantial proportion of these are middle aged. In Leicester, there were in 1981 about 2000 people over pensionable age, and in Birmingham well over 3000, who were born in the New Commonwealth or Pakistan, whereas in other parts of the country the numbers are neglible. See Table 8.1).
5. The whole emphasis of this book is upon the need to individualise assessment, care and planning for very old people, to combat against stereotyping. When to ageism is added racism, the danger of, at worst denigration, and at best condescension, is doubled. The religious, racial and cultural environment in which people have been brought up affects every facet of their daily lives. It is, therefore, essential for practitioners to have a raised awareness of the significance of these factors. It is as important in relation to a (say) solitary Ukranian as it is for a substantial concentration of (say) Afro-Caribbeans.

Table 8.1 Numbers of people of pensionable age born outside the UK, living in households whose head was born in the New Commonwealth and Pakistan. (From Barker, 1984.)

	East Africa	Caribbean	India	Bangladesh	New Commonwealth (other)	Pakistan	Total
Greater London							
Barnet	234	84	555	6	494	45	1418
Brent	430	929	853	5	352	66	2635
Bromley	16	63	297	3	109	25	513
Camden	18	144	235	27	539	25	988
Croydon	133	271	764	10	175	63	1416
Ealing	283	265	1358	4	264	106	2280
Enfield	73	126	246	7	549	14	1015
Greenwich	44	72	309	—	106	25	556
Hackney	21	836	252	8	400	17	1534
Hammersmith	24	350	201	5	193	19	792
Haringey	74	572	369	5	1104	18	2142
Harrow	338	74	497	4	136	46	1095
Hillingdon	61	20	323	—	71	26	501
Hounslow	202	65	671	3	153	73	1167
Islington	16	361	135	6	717	10	1245
Kens/Chelsea	26	215	259	9	217	30	756
Lambeth	59	1092	384	5	438	47	2025
Lewisham	27	521	236	2	190	13	989
Merton	49	134	375	4	138	56	756
Newham	160	282	512	5	104	49	1112
Redbridge	138	65	356	1	110	53	723
Southwark	21	444	105	5	373	15	963
Tower Hamlets	8	198	75	101	206	6	594
Waltham Forest	45	207	186	7	170	63	648
Wandsworth	116	628	488	10	295	52	1589
Westminster	21	314	252	10	382	31	1010
Metropolitan districts							
Manchester	46	362	224	5	102	89	828
Birmingham	181	1174	1327	60	138	344	3224
Coventry	82	63	531	7	50	31	764
Sandwell	21	177	530	7	24	16	775
Wolverhampton	33	289	643	2	20	16	1003
Bradford	35	67	359	15	26	169	671
Leeds	33	209	326	7	82	47	704
Shire counties							
Leicester	491	149	1311	6	55	25	2037
Nottingham	13	280	145	—	28	59	525

Norman (1985) lists and discusses the various ethnic minority groups under the headings of Jewish, Irish, Caribbean, Asian, European, Cypriot and Chinese. It is beyond the scope of this discussion to analyse and develop the many interesting points which she raises in connection with the specific groups. However, there are some matters which seem of particular importance to practitioners and which are not immediately self-evident.

One concerns the relationship of the past to the present. Literature on old age contains many references to the importance of talking about past experiences in work with elderly people. Sometimes, indeed, it seems a desperate bid on the part of the practitioner to find something interesting to relate to! At other times, it can be used constructively as part of an assessment process. Yet again, it is used as 'reminiscence therapy' in a more systematic fashion. For old people from ethnic minorities (even assuming that there is no language barrier), such interaction is often problematic. If practitioners have no knowledge of the countries from which old people have come, they have to travel imaginatively, not only back in time, but across oceans, if they are ever to glimpse the memories of the other. A particular sadness for some, perhaps especially Asian and Afro-Caribbeans, is that, contrary to wishes and even fantasies, most will not be able to return 'home' in their old age. For those whose decision to come to this country was primarily for the sake of employment, who long cherished an intention to return and who saw their hopes fading, memories will be bitter-sweet.

For another group, mainly Jews, but including others who have been persecuted, old age may bring a recurrence of terrifying memories. It has been observed that recollection of past experiences, repressed in middle years, may resurface in old age, when daily living pressures are less and inhibitions may be reduced. (This has been seen in war survivors.) It is, quite simply, impossible for us to enter imaginatively into the horrors of the holocaust – indeed, we would, in self-defence, turn away from such an endeavour. Yet practitioners will encounter old people who, as they sit now in comparative comfort and peace, have recurring visual memories of scenes of anguish and violence. However imperfectly, one has to seek to understand the impact of such horrors on present action and behaviour.

It is also important for practitioners to know just how culturally diverse may be those who we customarily link together. For example, Jewish settlers came from all over Europe and Asians living in Blackburn were found in 1978 to come from 17 different groups. Barker, as reported by Mays (1983) identified four main groups of current black and Asian elderly people. These were, firstly, 'the pioneers': the oldest Asian men who came to Britain in the 1930s and 1940s. Secondly, there were the early migrants, men from one part of India and women from the West Indies, now in their 60s and 70s. Many tended to feel left outside the mainstream of family life. A third group were the 'recent arrivals', parents and wives of the early migrants.

> In the case of the Asians, they are generally dependent on their children,
> have no pension entitlement and no role in the family since their children
> managed for a long period without them.   (Mays, 1983)

Lastly, there were the refugees, predominantly professional and managerial Asians who left East Africa in the late 1960s and early 1970s.

From such an analysis, it is immediately apparent how different will be the
needs of such elderly people. It also highlights the formidable difficulties in
constructing mechanisms for effective communication between the different
ethnic groups and those who fund or provide services.

A further dimension of experience concerns racism itself. This can be of two
kinds. Firstly, there is the direct personal unpleasantness and hostility which
may have been encountered because of their race. Discussion of this topic is
currently focused on those who are black or Asian, but this should not blind
us to the past experience of other old people, such as Jews in the 1930s when
Oswald Mosley's anti-semitic bands were on the march in London. Some,
particularly Asians, growing old in Britian today, have seen an increase in
racist attacks on their homes, a profoundly threatening manifestation of
antagonism. Less sinister, but symptomatic of our malaise, are the
derogatory remarks made to, or in front of, black elderly people. As one put it
(Lalljie,1983):

> The problem is they don't look on us as people, they look on us as black
> pensioners. They don't realise that we know we are black, and we are
> proud to be black. White people my age group is very selfish. They don't
> think we should even have a bus pass! I hear black people complain
> about some of the white pensioners who think black people should not
> have the things that are provided for pensioners.   (Lalljie,1983)

Thus, in addition to the general anxiety felt by so many old people in today's
society, black people may feel particularly vulnerable to abuse and even to
attack. However, problems arising from such overt racist attitudes are but a
small part of the whole.

Many practitioners who would be shocked at suggestions of overt racism
have come to realise to some extent the ways in which superficial assumptions and stereotypical views about people from different ethnic minorites
affect their attitudes and actions. These are matters for us all and are part of a
painful but essential process of self-awareness. They do not only affect individual interactions but also policy and practice in the provision of services. There
are also a wide range of social situations, in housing and employment for
example, in which certain groups have been the subject of discrimination. Yet
there has been too little concern amongst politicians and professionals to
redress the balance: there is sometimes active resistance to so doing.

All this adds up to a formidable package of disadvantage for people in ethnic
minorities, especially black and Asian, as they reach old age. The evidence on
this point is quite strong and demonstrates how disproportionately black

elderly people are trapped in the economic and social structured dependency which we discussed in Chapter 3. For example, as Norman (1985) points out research shows that

> Afro-Caribbeans and Asians in council properties tend to be put in high rise flats on unpopular estates, and those who have bought their own homes have been forced by availability and cost to take an old property in poor condition so that upkeep and heating are a struggle.

Severe housing problems are widespread in various ethnic communities and

> those who are old experience the same disadvantage, but they are often compounded by increasing disability, family tensions, loss of family support as younger people move out of the inner city, fear of racial harrassment and physical assault and social isolation.

Yet housing, as we have seen, is one of the most significant factors in the well-being of older people.

We have already noted that many old people who did not come to work here until they were adult, do not qualify for a full state pension and are thus more than usually dependent on the supplementary allowance, with all its means-tested corollaries. However, a specific and distressing aspect of hardship, potential and actual, in old age involves those who have come to this country since 1980 and whose relatives declared 'that he (sic) will maintain and accommodate his dependants without recourse to public funds in accommodation of his own or which he occupies himself'. Norman believes that this is a particular cause of fear and hardship for Chinese families with elderly dependants. If the provider fails to comply, he can be taken to court and his own right to stay in the UK may be threatened. Norman points out that

> there appears to be no official definition of 'public funds' and this gives rise to fear of using any free public service, including the National Health Service.

She cogently argues

> this clause has the effect of creating a group of elderly people in this country who are utterly without statutory right to housing, or financial benefits, and if they ask for such help they jeopardize their sponsor who will have broken his oath and thus committed a legal offence which can render him and his dependants liable to deportation. This condition would be a public scandal at any time: it is intolerable to have a group of elderly people in the country who may starve or die of exposure because they cannot ask for help. It is even more intolerable in a time of recession when, with the best will in the world, the sponsor may be unable to fulfil his commitments.

Whatever controls the state may choose to put on immigration and on definitions of dependants, there would seem to be an urgent need at least to clarify and limit this particular provision and preferably to abolish it altogether. It is quite unacceptable that its scope is not publicly defined and that changed circumstances and unforeseen difficulties may result in such misery and anxiety for families and old people. It is further indefensible for basic health provision to be in any way circumscribed, as in the case of an elderly Afro-Caribbean woman who returned to Jamaica because her family could not afford to pay for the spectacles, dentures and hearing aid which she required. Rules of this kind are so crude that they are bound to cause hardship and distress.

In fact it can be demonstrated that in almost every sphere of service provision, elements of deliberate racism, or racism by neglect and indifference, adversely affect old people in ethnic minority groups. This therefore places a serious responsibility on politicans, administrators and practitioners to address the particular elements which are their concern. As Norman (1985) remarks,

> although much has been said, very little has been done to remedy the situation except by the ethnic minority groups themselves. One reason for this may be that those who are most committed to eliminating ethnic disadvantage often know little about services for the elderly, while those concerned for the elderly may not be in the forefront of the fight for non-discrimination.

Inevitably when these matters are addressed, sensitive questions concerning the nature of the provision required will arise, in particular, of course, the extent to which ethnic groups should be separate from those of the white population. This matter is too complex and too fundamental to be discussed *en passant* here. It is one on which feelings run high and on which it is possible to hold entirely sincere but strongly differing views. In the context of this book, which is focused on the position of frail elderly people, it is perhaps less problematic. For it seems likely that many such old people will prefer, and feel safer in, the company of those whose appearance, behaviour and speech (even language) are familiar. Surely this should be respected. There will, of course, be logistical and practical problems in providing such an environment where the numbers concerned are small. But the attempt should be made, with one important proviso. It should not be regarded as self-evident that all such elderly people will want to be exclusively with their own ethnic group. This is ageist and racist. It will depend on individual attitudes and past experiences as well as the social climate which a particular social institution, such as a day centre, has created.

However, community care provision is not simply about 'getting people together'. It is about provision within the home. We are beginning to see consideration of domiciliary services tailored to meet the needs of ethnic groups, meals-on-wheels being an obvious example. Yet, as Norman reminds us, we must work urgently with the various ethnic groups to devise acceptable means of providing (such) services so that they can be developed, tried and tested before the many settlers now in their 60s and 70s become very old.

In matters as far reaching as these, it is easy to feel overwhelmed. Practitioners cannot and need not be all things to all people. It would seem, however, that they have three inescapable responsibilities. Firstly, workers in the caring professions must, through various alliances and pressure groups, work to change laws or regulations which are unjust or which have distressing consequences. They hold a particularly important position in such debates because of the 'grass roots' knowledge which they acquire of their workings. Secondly, as workers within a prescribed geographical area, they must take the trouble to find out what ethnic minority groups or individuals are living there and, broadly, their social circumstances. Thirdly, as workers within a particular service and with a particular role, they must address the impact, positive or negative, of that service and their work upon such old people and consider how they might be improved.

In all this they will need the help of representatives from the ethnic communities. They will, inevitably, pay the price for past neglect – their own and their predecessors. People will not be trusting and open. Why should they be? Nor may gratitude be more than institutional subservience. Yet, as Ahmed *et al.* (1986) point out:

> Treating people differently according to their real not their imagined needs or characteristics, is a recognition of the equal worth of different cultures; it may be a condition of equal treatment and a method of combatting racism.

Mental illness in old age

A second major issue in community care concerns the care of mentally ill and infirm old people. Much of the attention which this subject receives is focused on those suffering from dementia. This is understandable and we shall turn to this painful and disturbing topic later. However, it is important that this one disease of later years does not so dominate debate that the other matters of great significance are neglected.

Old people are subject to the same emotional and psychological disorders as anyone else. Their state of mind as adults, not as 'old people', should be assessed and their characteristic modes of behaviour and reaction over the years taken into account. In this way, one can begin to distinguish between long-standing patterns or recurring episodes and problems which appear to have arisen in old age.

There are two forms of mental illness in old age which merit special attention by practitioners who attend to their needs. The first concerns depression, the second dementia. The debate as to the part played by genetic or biochemical factors in depression rumbles on, as it does in relation to such psychiatric illnesses as schizophrenia. But the interaction of social and individual factors in depression is widely recognised as is the extent to which it is part of the 'human condition'. While in its most severe manifestations, it may show similarities to psychotic disorder, for most of us depression is part of life experience, to be borne and managed as best we may.

To distinguish, therefore, between depression as illness and depression as part of the human condition is not easy. In its most extreme forms, classical depression, marked by extreme guilt and despair in those who seem to have lost touch with external reality, does appear qualitatively different, although even that may be affected by the subjective world view of the others in the situation. For example, it can be argued that those whose profound depression is associated with the nuclear threat are more in touch with reality than the rest of us! Although such vivid and dramatic expressions of depression may be less common in very old age, deep sadness, which has many similarities to depression, may be a part of what Michael Key (Chapter 6) has described as 'appropriate suffering'. Whilst theories of disengagement in old age are now widely rejected as projecting a negative view of old age and encouraging ageism, we who are younger have to face the fact that such deep sadness may be part and parcel of the condition of old age. Old people have to accept that they have lost those they loved most and will never be able to replace them, that they will lose roles and functions which have been at the centre of their lives. For some, perhaps especially those who are reflective, there is a kind of existential depression which has to be borne and for which there is no remedy.

It is not widely realised that suicide rates rise steadily throughout life (Gray and Isaacs, 1979), with an especially sharp rise between the ages of 65 and 74. With men, the figure rises again in the last years of life but, interestingly, declines in women. On occasions, suicide may reflect a deliberate choice by someone who believes life has nothing more for them or who does not wish to live the rest of their lives as a burden to others. 'Rational' suicide, as euthanasia, are matters on which practitioners will hold strong and divergent views and the issues cannot be fully explored here. They are raised to point out the complexity of any discussion of depression in old age and of the distinction between 'normal' and 'abnormal' manifestations. However, there are other suicide attempts which arise from clinically disturbed mental states or chronic social isolation. Practitioners should not accept depression in old age as irremediable. On the contrary, there is a great deal that can be done through counselling, medication and increased social opportunities – in short, through approaching a very old person who appears depressed as one would anyone else but with an understanding of the special factors which may underlie in their condition.

Central to such work must be an appreciation of the impact of loss on old people's psychic state. It was Freud (1953) who first explored, with brilliant originality, the link between depression and loss, which is now so widely accepted. His analysis of 'melancholia' (clinical, pathological depression) suggested that the depressed person felt that he or she had lost, i.e. destroyed, a loved one through their own aggressive and hating impulses. This may or may not be associated with a recent loss, for example through death, in external reality. Those who work with the bereaved will often see evidence of such feelings of guilt even in relatively normal grief reactions and it is widely accepted that the greater the ambivalence about the person who has died, the more likely it is that such reactions will occur. The literature on such matters is now extensive, although, as discussed in Chapter 1, it has been insufficiently related to the situations and characteristics of very old people. For example, Rowlings (1981) points out that 'there is some evidence to suggest that a pattern of grief may be slightly different in old people'. She cites Gramlich (1973) suggesting that

> inhibited or chronic grief may be common amongst elderly people. . . . The significance of inhibited grief is that, whilst appearing subdued, it is long lasting and may well be associated with physical or psychological symptoms. . . . Chronic grief is associated with intense feeling over a longer time span than is found in typical grief and may give rise to hostility, suspicion or apathy.

One of the complicating factors in reactions to bereavement, especially to the loss of a partner, is that old people may have fewer opportunities to share their feelings about it with others. So as Rowlings put it, they may become 'stuck' in their grief, 'unable to establish an equilibrium'.

As has already been stressed, multiple losses are of particular significance in old age. Old people's adaptability is remarkable but the cumulative impact of different kinds of loss in creating depression is considerable – partners, relatives, friends, as well as the loss of bodily function, role and status. Nor should one forget the importance of pets and animals in the daily lives of some old people and therefore the sense of loss when they die. Although this can all too easily be sentimentalised, and therefore ridiculed, it is important to acknowledge that to be bereft of the company and comfort of a living being, especially when one is isolated and lonely, is a cause of appropriate grief.

It is therefore hardly possible to overestimate the significance of loss in assessments of elderly people's state of mind. Obviously, this can have a direct bearing on plans made for and with them for the future. In particular, expressed wishes to move house and perhaps to enter residential care should be treated with reserve when they occur soon after such a loss. Moreover, the fact that someone's depression seems understandable, given what they have had to endure, does not mean that nothing can be done to relieve its more distressing symptoms. This all points to the need for specialist appraisal.

Working with old people who appear depressed presents a formidable but very interesting challenge because it requires us to ask searching questions of ourselves about our attitudes to this last stage of life. On the one hand, we must acknowledge the inescapable sadness of it. As with all depressed people, that may enable us to stay alongside, to offer the wordless comfort of another human being who is willing to share some of the pain. On the other hand, as with physical illness in old age, we should be keen to explore modes of intervention which may shift the balance from sadness to hope in the lives of old people, above all which will give new meaning and purpose to daily life. Gray and Isaacs (1979), reporting an earlier study on suicide in old people, comment that 'the tone of many suicide notes is eloquent of the feeling of worthlessness and being a burden'. As a society, we should be deeply ashamed when old people kill (or indeed severely neglect) themselves because they feel that no one cares any more whether they live or die and we have done little or nothing to prove them wrong.

We turn now to that most formidable mental illness of old age – dementia. As Norman (1987) remarks,

> if service provision is to be properly planned, a more up to date and sophisticated epidemiological study of the incidence of dementia than that done in Newcastle in the 1960s is urgently needed.

However, Norman's analysis of the situation starkly reveals the dimensions of the problem which we face.

> It is however clear that the Newcastle researchers were right in finding that incidence rises very steeply with age. They estimated 2.8 per cent of sufferers in the 71–74 age group, 5.5 per cent in the 75–79 age group and 22 per cent in the over 80s. The number of people in the UK aged 80 plus is expected to increase by nearly 300,000 between the year of writing (1986) and 2001. If 22 per cent are dementia sufferers, there will be an increase of 66,000 cases in this age group alone and even if 90 per cent of them can be looked after in ordinary housing or integrated residential care (an optimistic estimate) we will need 6,600 more long stay beds for dementia suffers in their 80s by 2001 than we have at present, and current provision is inadequate both in quantity and quality. These figures drive home both the importance and urgency of getting our plans and our models for longstay provision right as quickly as possible.

Dementia is a disease in which the cells of the brain are progressively destroyed. There are two main kinds: Alzheimer's disease, in which the brain itself is diseased, and multi-infarct dementia, caused by frequent minor strokes which cut off the blood supply to the brain. It is important that these should not be confused with forgetfulness and other minor 'muddles' to which the very old are prone, nor with sudden bouts of confusion, often due to infection or toxic states. Although the way in which dementia is managed may to an extent affect people's behaviour, the condition is not socially induced, as some earlier sociological writings (Meacher, 1972) seemed to imply.

Gray and Isaacs (1979) give a useful account of common manifestations of brain failure of which they give five illustrative cases. These are:

1. 'the burned out kettle', in which the person shows 'diminished vigilance, accompanied by failure to register recent events, especially in relation to self initiated acts. Neither the error nor the consequences are perceived';
2. 'the living dead', in which 'the patient speaks of her long dead mother as though she were still alive . . . she fails to distinguish between reverie and reality';
3. the '28 lb of sugar', in which 'the patient comes home with 28 lb of sugar she does not need. . . . In this, the patient is persevering in a familiar behaviour pattern which has now outlived its former usefulness and relevance';
4. 'concealed underwear. . . . The patient who has always been clean and fastidious, soils underwear with urine and faeces'. Of this Gray and Isaacs comment:

   > Few symptoms give more offence or cause more distress than this one. The explanation is to be found in the patient's image of her own ego. She sees herself, as she always has done, as a clean, continent and responsible person. When she finds the soiled underwear she has little or no recollection of having soiled it, and she cannot conceive of it as having been soiled by herself. She therefore 'detaches' the garment, soilage and all, from her body and from her body image.

5. Lastly, Gray and Isaacs describe 'wandering'; they suggest that this may be an 'urge for voyage and discovery unfulfilled', or that 'the wanderer is restlessly searching for her lost world'.

Such descriptions will be recognised by those who have worked with or cared for old people with dementia, and it is valuable to have both the analysis and their suggestions of management. However, they also highlight the extent to which the disease remains a mystery and its symptoms and progress often baffling to those who care for the old people. For example, the explanations of wandering given by Gray and Isaacs are not altogether convincing. Nor is it clear how far the vagaries of behaviour are explicable solely in terms of the damage done to various parts of the brain which control certain functions, and how far the brain damage may disinhibit and thus cause feelings and behaviour to be displayed which in earlier years were controlled. The concealed underwear is a case in point. Those of us who have worked in the field of child welfare are familiar with the emotionally disturbed 'deprived' child who does likewise but for whose behaviour physiological explanations do not appear appropriate. Is there a link between the two?

While those who work with dementing old people will find it distressing, there is no reason to find it dull. It raises intriguing psychological questions. Concentration on those most severely demented, and for whom environmental management may be the only effective intervention, should not cause us to neglect many others less seriously impaired but who need help in specific aspects of their lives. (Some of whom have painful insight in to their condition and fears and anxieties about the future.) Above all, as Levin *et al.* (1983) have shown so well, those who care for this group of elderly people deserve and urgently need our most imaginative responses in devising supportive strategies. There are some parallels between dementia and AIDS in the sense that we confront diseases at present incurable, which affect a significant and growing number of the population and which cause great distress to carers, albeit for very different reasons. Is it too much to hope that some of the same energy will go into the response to dementia as is evident with the newly discovered AIDS?

This group of people, then, pose some of the most serious difficulties for 'care in the community', whether formal or informal. Indeed, it is generally accepted that it is the seriously demented who may require the lion's share of the future residential provision, since the alternative community support may simply not be sufficient to maintain such old people in safety and decency at home, or the burden on their relatives may be intolerable.

However, hundreds of thousands of old people with this disease will live in private households. The disease is variable in its rate of progress, but it is measured in years rather than months. Long before its final phase, in which, especially for those who live alone, residential care may be the only practicable solution, practitioners should be appropriately involved in devising structures of support and offering advice on management.

There is a wide range of provision available which, if properly coordinated, can do much to relieve both patient and carer. As Arie (1985) has shown, practitioners need to draw on a variety of services from different sources, taking account of the notorious unevenness of their availability in different areas. Broadly, these may be categorised as follows: forms of support, such as day care, outside the home; help with financial affairs; domiciliary support – such as home helps and practical measures to ensure greater safety; support to carers through, for example, relatives groups; medication and residential care. These add up to quite an impressive array with social, rather than medical, assistance to the fore. It remains a taxing problem to make such provision adequately for two reasons. Firstly, demand outstrips supply. Secondly, it is not easy to make available the particular forms of support or intervention which an old person or their carer may need or want. Arie concludes:

> Old people with failing brains have three main needs: security because their capacity to function physically far outstrips their capacity to adapt to change; stimulation because dementia, especially when accompanied by restricted mobility and sensory privation in the form of deafness or blindness, makes the world a frightening and lonely place, in which withdrawal and apathy may be the way of least resistance; and patience because old people are slow, but time and again they astonish one by their capacity to 'get there in the end'. . . . Of course, these needs are not

confined to the demented elderly. They are among the basic needs of all of us, but the disabilities of the demented make their needs more urgent, and their lack of inhibit'on may make more direct the efforts to satisfy them. The attention seeking behaviour of old people, their wandering and incontinence, may become at least partly intelligible, and so perhaps more manageable, if seen against the background of these needs.

What the Barclay Committee (1982) describes as 'social care planning' is vital in the care of old people with dementia living alone. The construction of packages of care, discussed earlier, is integral to this. They nearly always require inputs from a variety of statutory, voluntary and informal sources. Their reliability is critical, for the failure of one element may have grave repercussions. They have to be subjected to systematic review, as the condition of the old person deteriorates. In effect, these packages are the key to effective policies of community care for mentally infirm old people. In the paper by Addison (1984) the author notes the importance of developing ways of dealing with anxiety in carers – formal and informal. Although this has general applicability, it has special relevance to neighbours and other locally involved people who are concerned about confused old people at home alone. Dementia, above all, creates anxiety in carers because of the element of unpredictability and consequently risk. Those who feel themselves becoming too involved without adequate backing from the professionals may withdraw altogether.

Because dementia is a slow progressive disorder, it creates in those who care for and work with such people very difficult dilemmas concerning the autonomy of the person concerned, to which reference was earlier made in more general terms. Most living in the community still have the capacity to manage aspects of daily living but these capacities diminish, sometimes very steadily and gradually, sometimes in spurts, after periods of relative stability. When do the various elements in independent living get taken over by other people, notably the management of money and bills, cooking, cleaning and self care? At a certain point, the right of old people to live their own lives can work against their interests, not simply in matters like risk or self-neglect, but in the reactions of others to their appearance or household. Take, for example, the apparently trivial matter of removing facial hair in old women. When that is neglected, it changes the appearance and presents, especially to children, a negative image, which can have repercussions in the form of teasing and vandalism. It is too facile to say 'if she doesn't want to bother, why should we?'. Similarly, once a house begins to smell, fewer people will be willing to call and isolation is increased. Possibly the best way to approach this is to seek to understand what dimensions of daily living give the person most satisfaction or pleasure and to devise daily living strategies which preserve these as long as possible.

The record of the statutory sector in supporting those who care for the mentally infirm in their own homes has not been good, but it is fair to say that this subject has received much more attention from the professionals in the last 5–10 years. Society generally has become much more aware of, and sensitive to, their plight and there have been a number of moving programmes and articles on the subject. We have earlier discussed the position of those who tend old people and the assumptions which have been made about 'women's work'. Caring for those with dementia raises more acutely and dramatically tensions and dilemmas which may be present in other forms of care. This is because the demands made are multifarious and the strain greater. It is in the nature of the illness that such people cannot be left much by themselves; that their care requires watchfulness to avoid danger; that some of their daily habits are distasteful; and that communication with them becomes less and less rewarding. Of this last, the despairing cry is frequently heard: 'she is not my mother anymore, she is dead to me already'. Although such comments may only be made in the last stages of the illness and, in some cases, such a stage is never reached, it does highlight an issue which practitioners must face in offering support in the community. The underlying assumption in such work has been that support is designed to maintain such old people at home with their relatives until it is absolutely impossible to continue. Yet there are fine judgements to be made as to when that point is reached. The intense stress, emotional and physical, which carers experience can, if insufficiently acknowledged, lead to breakdown and have far-reaching consequences for their later state of mind. A situation in which a carer has to cry for attention by, for example, expressing to practitioners fears that she will abuse an old person if not offered relief, is humiliating. It is sad, indeed, if it is felt that this is the only way to get help. One must further recognise that if the old person has lost the capacity to relate meaningfully to the carer, there may be a sense in which the relationship, as a kind of life long contract, has been broken. What may then be needed is help to give up, rather than maintain, care.

Such work with individuals, however, takes place in a context of severe shortage of suitable provision and pressure on practitioners to delay admission to residential care as long as possible. Development of long-stay provision is a critical part of effective work with carers. Table 8.2 outlines the present position.

As Norman (1987) points out, 'private proprietors are as yet providing specialist care on a fairly limited scale'. Although private homes which are not classified as specialist have a substantial proportion of confused residents, it is clear that relatively few are staffed or have the skills to contain severely demented people. Moreover, the distribution of both nursing and rest homes which offer this kind of care is very varied across the country.

So far as NHS is concerned, '70% of longstay provision is still based in traditional psychiatric hospitals, while a mere 5% is in the local units which are now officially recognised as the proper place for such provision' (Norman,

1987). Although many hospitals have made strenuous efforts to improve the quality of life in such long-stay wards, many have, for the old people and for their relatives, long-standing stigmatising associations and some today fall short of acceptable standards. For example, can one justify the persisting problems in ensuring that patients get their own clothes back from the laundry? Local authority designated specialist care provides a mere 12 per cent of the places, although, as in the private sector, many of those in their care suffer from a substantial degree of infirmity. Again, the provision is very patchy.

Thus, any discussion of community care for this group of people, whose care and management is so difficult, has to take cognisance of the serious deficiencies in available alternatives. This places both carers and practitioners in painful and stressful predicaments and makes talk of 'choice' ring hollow. It may be, however, that on occasions an honest acknowledgement by a worker to a carer that the case for residential care is overwhelming will at least relieve some of the guilt so commonly experienced by the carer.

This discussion has concentrated upon two of the most common manifestations of mental illness in old age – depression and dementia. There is, of course, much more to be said about the issue generally. The intention here is to place mental infirmity in old age high on the agenda in any consideration of community care. It presents grave and sometimes intractable difficulties. But it also offers practitioners a remarkable opportunity to make effective interventions of inestimable importance to the parties, including the carers, whether through the cure or alleviation of depression or through the effective management of the disabilities of the demented.

Table 8.2 Specialist provision in England. (Data from Norman, 1987.)

National Health Service	Traditional hospital	Geriatric hospital	District general hospital	Local units	Total	%
	17 482	3 593	2 258	1 272	24 605	79
Local authority	Shires	Metropolitan boroughs	London boroughs			
	2 169	1 069	751		3 989	12
Private	Nursing homes	Residential homes	Voluntary residential homes			
	1 352	1 032	122		2 506	8
				Grand total:	31 000	

Postscript

'You ask me what old people need, they need the same as everybody else. They want to feel wanted. They want to feel when they wake up in the morning that it's going to matter to someone that they live another day. Nothing about being old that makes us special. I'm still the same person I always was, a bit uglier and more awkward than I was, a bit more bad-tempered, but I'm still me.'

'Life isn't about what I want, what I'm going to get. It's as much about what I can give. That way you get repaid a hundredfold; but it doesn't come in material things. You can't see it wrapped up in silver paper; it comes through the heart and the feelings and the joy people can *give* each other.'

(*In* Seabrook, 1980)

An ethic built on caring is thought by some to be tenderminded. It does involve construction of an ideal from the fact and memory of tenderness. The ethical sentiment itself requires a prior natural sentiment of caring and a willingness to sustain tenderness. But there is no assumption of innate human goodness . . .

When we accept honestly our loves, our innate ferocity, our capacity for hate, we may use all this as information in building the safe-guards and alarms that must be part of the ideal. We know better what we must work toward, what we must prevent. . . .

Instead of hiding from our natural impulses and pretending that we can achieve goodness through lofty abstractions, we accept what is there – all of it – and use what we have already assessed as good to control that which is not-good.

Everything depends, then, upon the will to be good, to remain in caring relation to the other. How may we help ourselves and each other to sustain this will?

(Noddings, 1984)

We must stop cheating: the whole meaning of our life is in question in the future that is waiting for us. If we do not know what we are going to be, we cannot know what we are. Let us recognise ourselves in this old man or in that old woman. It must be done if we are to take upon ourselves the entirety of our human state. And when it is done we will no longer acquiesce in the misery of old age; we will no longer be indifferent, because we shall feel concerned, as indeed we are.

(Simone de Beauvoir, 1977)

References

Books specially recommended are indicated with an asterisk.

Abrams, M. (1978). *Beyond Three Score and Ten, 1st Report.* Age Concern England, Surrey.

Abrams, M. (1980). *Beyond Three Score and Ten, 2nd Report.* Age Concern England, Surrey.

Abrams, S. and Marsden, D. (1986). *Companions, Liberators, Intruders and Cuckoos in the Nest. A sociology of informal caring relationships over the life cycle.* Paper to British Sociological Conference at Loughborough (University of Essex).

*Addison, C. (1984). *A report on collaboration in relation to the frail elderly.* Wandsworth Borough Council, London.

Ahmed, S., Cheetham, J. and Small, J. (1986). *Social Work with Black Children and their Families.* Batsford, London.

Allan, G. (1986). Friendship and care for elderly people. *Ageing and Society,* **6**, 1: 1–12.

Arber, S., Evandrou, M., Gilbert, C.N. and Dale, H. (1986). *Gender, Carers and Receipt of Formal Services by the Elderly Disabled.* Paper to British Sociological Conference at Loughborough (University of Surrey).

Arie, T. (1985). Dementia in the elderly: Management. In *Medicine in Old Age.* British Medical Association, London.

Audit Commission (1985). *Managing Social Services for the Elderly More Effectively.* HMSO, London.

Audit Commission (1986). *Making a Reality of Community Care.* HMSO, London.

Barclay Committee (1982). *Social Workers: Their roles and tasks* (Report). National Institute of Social Work, London.

Barker, J. (1984). *Black and Asian Old People in Britain*. Age Concern England, Surrey.

Barrowclough, C. and Fleming, I. (1986). *Goal Planning with Elderly People: Making Plans to Meet Individual Needs*. Manchester University Press, Manchester.

Barton, R. (1959). *Institutional Neurosis*. John Wright & Sons, Bristol.

Bettelheim, B. (1970). *The Informed Heart*. Paladin Books, London.

Bhalla, A. and Blakemore, K. (1981). *Elders of the Minority Ethnic Groups*. Affor, Birmingham.

Booth, T.A. (1985). *Home Truths: Old People's Homes and the Outcome of Care*. Gower Publishing, Hants.

Bornat, J., Phillipson, C. and Ward, S. (1985). *A Manifesto for Old Age*. Pluto Press, London.

*Bowlby, J. (1979). *The Making and Breaking of Affectional Bonds*. Tavistock Publications, London.

Bradshaw, J. (1972). The concept of need. *New Society*, 30th March.

*Bulmer, M. (Ed.) (1986). *Neighbours: The Work of Philip Abrams*. Cambridge University Press, Cambridge.

Bulmer, M. (1987). *The Social Basis of Community Care*. Allen & Unwin, London.

*Burns, B. and Phillipson, C. (1986). *Drugs, Ageing and Society*. Croom Helm, Kent.

Challis, D. and Davies, B. (1987). *Case Management in Community Care*. Gower Publishing, Hants.

*Cloke, C. (1983). *Old Age Abuse in the Domestic Setting*. Age Concern England, Surrey.

Curtis Committee (1946). *Report of the Care of Children Committee*. Cmnd. 6922. HMSO, London.

De Beauvoir, S. (1977). *Old Age*. Penguin, Middlesex.

Department of Health and Social Security (1981). *Census 1981. National Report*. DHSS, London.

Department of Health and Social Security (1985/1986). *Reform of Social Security. Programme for change*, Cmnd. 9518. *Programme for action*, Cmnd. 9519. HMSO, London.

Department of Health and Social Security (1987). *Public Support for Residential Care*. (The Firth Report). DHSS, London.

Drabble, M. (1980). *The Middle Ground*. Weidenfeld & Nicolson, London.

Eastman, M. (1984). *Old Age Abuse*. Age Concern England, Surrey.

Equal Opportunities Commission (1980). *The experience of caring for elderly and handicapped dependants: A survey report*. EOC, Manchester.

Equal Opportunities Commission (1982). *Caring for the elderly and handicapped: Community care policies and women's lives*. EOC, Manchester.

*Equal Opportunities Commission (1982). *Who cares for the carers?*

Opportunities for those caring for the elderly and handicapped. EOC, Manchester.

*Equal Opportunities Commission (1984). *Carers and services: A comparison of men and women caring for dependent elderly people.* EOC, Manchester.

Evers, V. (1984). Old women's self perception of dependency and some implications for service provision. *Journal of Epidemiology and Community Health,* **38**: 306–9.

Family Policy Studies Centre (1984). *An ageing population.* Fact Sheet. Open University Press, Milton Keynes.

Fillenbaum, G. (1985). *The Well-being of the Elderly: Approaches to Multidimensional Assessment.* World Health Organization, HMSO, London.

*Finch, J. and Groves, D. (1983). *A Labour of Love. Women, Work and Caring.* Routlege & Kegan Paul, London.

Freud, S. (1953). *Collected Papers, Volume IV. VIII Mourning and Melancholia.* Hogarth Press, London.

Giddens, A. (1984). *The Constitution of Society: Outline of the Theory of Structuration.* Polity Press, Cambridge.

Goffman, E. (1961). *Asylums.* Anchor Books; Doubleday, Coventry.

Goldberg, M. and Connelly, N. (1982). *The Effectiveness of Social Care for the Elderly.* Heinemann, London.

Gramlich, E. (1973). Recognition and management of grief in elderly patients. *Readings in Gerontology,* V. Brandt and M. Brown (Eds). pp. 105–10.

*Gray, B. and Isaacs, B. (1979). *Care of the Elderly Mentally Infirm.* Tavistock Publications, London.

*Greengross, S. (1986). *The Law and Vulnerable Elderly People.* Age Concern England, Surrey.

*Griffiths, R. (1988). *Community Care: Agenda for Action. A report to the Secretary of State for Social Services.* HMSO, London.

Herbert, G. (1972). The Flower. In *Oxford Book of Religious Verse,* Gardner (Ed.). Oxford University Press, Oxford.

Home Life: A Code of Practice for Residential Care. Working Party Report. (1984). Centre for Policy on Ageing, London.

House of Commons (1985). *Social Services Committee, Volume I. Community Care.* HMSO, London.

Ignatieff, M. (1984). *The Needs of Strangers.* Chatto & Windus, London.

Isaacs, B. (1981). Ageing of the doctor. In *The Impact of Ageing,* D. Hobman (Ed.). Croom Helm, Kent.

Jerrome, D. (1981). The significance of friendship for women in later life. *Ageing and Society,* **1**, 2: 175–98.

Kane, R. and Kane, R. (1981). *Assessing the Elderly.* Lexington Books, USA.

*Key, M. (1985). *Critical Social Work for Healthy Dying. Warwick Critical Studies No. 3.* Department of Applied Social Studies, University of Warwick.

King, R., Raynes, N. and Tizard, J. (1971). *Patterns of Residential Care.* Routledge & Kegan Paul, London.

Lalljie, R. (1983). *Black Elders.* Nottingham County Council Social Services Department, Nottingham.

*Levin, E., Sinclair, I. and Gorbach, P. (1983). *The Supporters of Confused Elderly Persons at Home.* National Institute for Social Work, London.

Lewis, J. and Meredith B. (1988). *Daughters who Care.* Tavistock Publications, London.

McCullough, A. (1981). What do we mean by development in old age? *Ageing and Society,* **1**, 2: 229–46.

*MacDonald, B. and Rich, C. (1984). *Look me in the Eye. Old Women, Ageing and Ageism.* Women's Press, London.

*Marris, P. (1974). *Loss and Change.* Routledge & Kegan Paul, London.

*Matthews, S. (1979). *The Social World of Old Women: Management of Self-identity.* Sage Publications, London.

Mays, N. (1983). Elderly Asians in Britain. *Ageing and Society,* **3**, 1: 44–70.

Meacher, M. (1972). *Taken for a ride.* Longman, Essex.

Menzies, I.E.P. (1960). A case study in the functioning of social systems as a defence against anxiety. *Human Relations,* **13**

Midwinter, E. (1986). *Caring for Cash: The issue of private domiciliary care.* Centre for Policy on Ageing, London.

National Institute for Social Work (1988). *A Positive Choice* (The Wagner Report). NISW, London

Nissel, M. and Bonnerjea, L. (1982). *Family Care of the Handicapped Elderly: Who Pays?* Policy Studies Institute, London.

Noddings, N. (1984). *Caring: A feminine approach to ethics and moral education.* University of California Press, California.

*Norman, A. (1980). *Rights and Risk.* (National Corporation for the Care of Old People) Centre for Policy on Ageing, London.

*Norman, A. (1985). *Triple Jeopardy: Growing Old in a Second Homeland.* Centre for Policy on Ageing, London.

Norman, A. (1987). *Severe Dementia: The Provision of Long Stay Care.* Centre for Policy on Ageing

Office of Population Censuses and Surveys (1980). *General Household Survey.* OPCS, London.

Oliver, J. (1986). Open letter in *Social Work Today,* 11th August.

Parker, R. (1981). Tending and Social Policy. In *A New Look at the Social Services,* E.M. Goldberg and S. Hatch (Eds). Policy Studies Institute, London.

*Parkes, C.M. (1986). *Bereavement: Studies of Grief in Adult Life.* Pelican Books, London.

Pattie, A.H. and Gilleard, C.J. (1979). *Manual for the Clifton Assessment Procedures for the Elderly (CAPE).* Hodder & Stoughton Educational, Sevenoaks.

*Phillipson, C. and Walker, A. (1986). *Ageing and Social Policy.* Gower Publications, Hants.

Priestley, J.B. (1974). In *San Francisco Chronicle Examiner*.

*Rowlings, C. (1981). *Social Work with Elderly People*. Allen & Unwin, London.

Royal College of Physicians (1984). Medication for the elderly. *Journal of the Royal College of Physicians*, **18**, 1: 7–17.

Seabrook, J. (1980). *The Way We Are: Old people talk about themselves*. Age Concern England, Surrey.

Sengstock, M. and Liang, J. (1982). *Identifying and Characterising Elder Abuse*. Institute of Gerontology, Wayne State University, Michigan.

*Sinclair, I. (1987). *Homes for the Elderly. Independent Review of Residential Care*. National Institute of Social Work, London.

Skegg, D., Doll, R. and Perry, J. (1986). The Use of Medicines in General Practice. *British Medical Journal* **(i)**: 1561–3.

Stevenson, O. (1986). *Women in Old Age*. Inaugural Lecture, Nottingham University.

Stevenson, O. (1988). Frail elderly people in poverty. In *Public Issues: Private Pain, Poverty, Social Work and Social Policy*, S. Becker and S. MacPherson (Eds). Care Matters, London.

Taylor, H. (1986). *Growing Old Together*. Centre for Policy on Ageing, London.

Tinker, A. (1984). *Staying at Home: Helping Elderly People*. Department of the Environment, London.

Townsend, P. (1964). *The Last Refuge*. Routledge & Kegan Paul, London.

Townsend, P. (1981). The structured dependency of the elderly. *Ageing and Society*, **1**, 1: 5–28.

Ungerson, C. (1983). In *A Labour of Love: Women Work and Caring*, J. Finch and D. Groves (Eds). Routledge & Kegan Paul, London.

Ungerson, C. (1983). Women and caring: Skills, tasks and taboos. In *The Public and the Private*, E. Gamarnakow, D. Morgan, J. Purvis and T. Taylorson (Eds). Heinemann, London.

Van Deurzen-Smith, E. (1984). Existential Therapy. In *Individual Therapy in Britain*, W. Dryden (Ed.). Harper & Row, London.

Wagner, G. (1988). *A Positive Choice*. National Institute for Social Work; London.

Walker, A. (1981). Towards a political economy of old age. *Ageing and Society*, **1**, 1: 73–94.

*Weaver, T., Willcocks, D. and Kellaher, L. (1985). *The Business of Care: A study of private residential homes for old people*. Centre for Enviornmental and Social Studies in Ageing, Polytechnic of North London.

Wenger, C. (1984). *The Supportive Network*. Allen & Unwin, London.

*Wheeler, R. (1982). Staying Put: A new development in policy. *Ageing and Society*, **2**, 3: 299–330.

Wicks, M. (1978). *Old and Cold*. Heinemann, London.

*Willcocks, D., Peace, S. and Kellaher, L. (1987). *Private Lives in Public Places*. Tavistock Publications, London.

Williamson, J. (1981). Screening, surveillance and case findings. In *Health Care of the Elderly*, T. Arie (Ed.), pp. 194–213. Croom Helm, Kent.

Woods, R. and Britton, P. (1985). *Clinical Psychology with the Elderly*. Croom Helm, Kent.

*Worden, J.W. (1983). *Grief Counselling and Grief Therapy*. Tavistock Publications, London.

Index